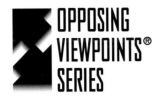

OPPOSING VIEWPOINTS® SERIES

The Opioid Crisis

Erica Grove, Book Editor

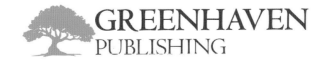

GREENHAVEN PUBLISHING

Published in 2023 by Greenhaven Publishing, LLC
2544 Clinton Street,
Buffalo NY 14224

Articles in Greenhaven Publishing anthologies are often edited for length to meet page
requirements. In addition, original titles of these works are changed to clearly present
the main thesis and to explicitly indicate the author's opinion. Every effort is made to
ensure that Greenhaven Publishing accurately reflects the original intent of the authors.
Every effort has been made to trace the owners of the copyrighted material.

Cover image: Leigh A. Williams/Shutterstock.com

Library of Congress CataloginginPublication Data

Names: Grove, Erica M., editor.
Title: The opioid crisis / Erica Grove, book editor
Description: First edition | New York : Greenhaven Publishing, 2023. |
  Series: Opposing viewpoints | Includes bibliographical references and
  index. | Audience: Ages 15+ | Audience: Grades 10-12 | Summary:
  "Anthology of essays addressing the opioid crisis in the US"-- Provided
  by publisher.
Identifiers: LCCN 2022018027 | ISBN 9781534509061 (library binding) | ISBN
  9781534509054 (paperback)
Subjects: LCSH: Opioid abuse--Juvenile literature. | Drug abuse--Juvenile
  literature.
Classification: LCC RC568.O45 O7544 2023 | DDC 362.29/3--dc23/eng/20220505
LC record available at https://lccn.loc.gov/2022018027

Manufactured in the United States of America

Website: http://greenhavenpublishing.com

> "Congress shall make no law ... abridging the freedom of speech, or of the press."

First Amendment to the U.S. Constitution

The basic foundation of our democracy is the First Amendment guarantee of freedom of expression. The Opposing Viewpoints series is dedicated to the concept of this basic freedom and the idea that it is more important to practice it than to enshrine it.

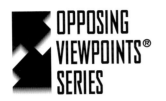

The Opioid Crisis

Other Books of Related Interest

Opposing Viewpoints Series

Big Pharma and Drug Pricing
Harm Reduction
Mass Incarceration

At Issue Series

The Opioid Crisis
Universal Health Care
Vaping

Current Controversies Series

America's Mental Health Crisis
Homelessness and Street Crime
Medical Use of Illicit Drugs

Contents

Chapter 3: Who Is Responsible for the Opioid Crisis, and Can They Be Held Accountable?

Chapter 4: Can the Opioid Crisis Be Stopped?

The Importance of Opposing Viewpoints

Perhaps every generation experiences a period in time in which the populace seems especially polarized, starkly divided on the important issues of the day and gravitating toward the far ends of the political spectrum and away from a consensus-facilitating middle ground. The world that today's students are growing up in and that they will soon enter into as active and engaged citizens is deeply fragmented in just this way. Issues relating to terrorism, immigration, women's rights, minority rights, race relations, health care, taxation, wealth and poverty, the environment, policing, military intervention, the proper role of government—in some ways, perennial issues that are freshly and uniquely urgent and vital with each new generation—are currently roiling the world.

If we are to foster a knowledgeable, responsible, active, and engaged citizenry among today's youth, we must provide them with the intellectual, interpretive, and critical-thinking tools and experience necessary to make sense of the world around them and of the all-important debates and arguments that inform it. After all, the outcome of these debates will in large measure determine the future course, prospects, and outcomes of the world and its peoples, particularly its youth. If they are to become successful members of society and productive and informed citizens, students need to learn how to evaluate the strengths and weaknesses of someone else's arguments, how to sift fact from opinion and fallacy, and how to test the relative merits and validity of their own opinions against the known facts and the best possible available information. The landmark series Opposing Viewpoints has been providing students with just such critical-thinking skills and exposure to the debates surrounding society's most urgent contemporary issues for many years, and it continues to serve this essential role with undiminished commitment, care, and rigor.

The key to the series's success in achieving its goal of sharpening students' critical-thinking and analytic skills resides in its title—

Opposing Viewpoints. In every intriguing, compelling, and engaging volume of this series, readers are presented with the widest possible spectrum of distinct viewpoints, expert opinions, and informed argumentation and commentary, supplied by some of today's leading academics, thinkers, analysts, politicians, policy makers, economists, activists, change agents, and advocates. Every opinion and argument anthologized here is presented objectively and accorded respect. There is no editorializing in any introductory text or in the arrangement and order of the pieces. No piece is included as a "straw man," an easy ideological target for cheap point-scoring. As wide and inclusive a range of viewpoints as possible is offered, with no privileging of one particular political ideology or cultural perspective over another. It is left to each individual reader to evaluate the relative merits of each argument— as he or she sees it, and with the use of ever-growing critical-thinking skills—and grapple with his or her own assumptions, beliefs, and perspectives to determine how convincing or successful any given argument is and how the reader's own stance on the issue may be modified or altered in response to it.

This process is facilitated and supported by volume, chapter, and selection introductions that provide readers with the essential context they need to begin engaging with the spotlighted issues, with the debates surrounding them, and with their own perhaps shifting or nascent opinions on them. In addition, guided reading and discussion questions encourage readers to determine the authors' point of view and purpose, interrogate and analyze the various arguments and their rhetoric and structure, evaluate the arguments' strengths and weaknesses, test their claims against available facts and evidence, judge the validity of the reasoning, and bring into clearer, sharper focus the reader's own beliefs and conclusions and how they may differ from or align with those in the collection or those of their classmates.

Research has shown that reading comprehension skills improve dramatically when students are provided with compelling, intriguing, and relevant "discussable" texts. The subject matter of these collections could not be more compelling, intriguing, or urgently relevant to today's students and the world they are poised to inherit. The anthologized articles and the reading and discussion questions that are included with them also provide the basis for stimulating, lively, and passionate classroom debates. Students who are compelled to anticipate objections to their own argument and identify the flaws in those of an opponent read more carefully, think more critically, and steep themselves in relevant context, facts, and information more thoroughly. In short, using discussable text of the kind provided by every single volume in the Opposing Viewpoints series encourages close reading, facilitates reading comprehension, fosters research, strengthens critical thinking, and greatly enlivens and energizes classroom discussion and participation. The entire learning process is deepened, extended, and strengthened.

For all of these reasons, Opposing Viewpoints continues to be exactly the right resource at exactly the right time—when we most need to provide readers with the critical-thinking tools and skills that will not only serve them well in school but also in their careers and their daily lives as decision-making family members, community members, and citizens. This series encourages respectful engagement with and analysis of opposing viewpoints and fosters a resulting increase in the strength and rigor of one's own opinions and stances. As such, it helps make readers "future ready," and that readiness will pay rich dividends for the readers themselves, for the citizenry, for our society, and for the world at large.

Introduction

> "Opioids reach every part of society:
> blue collar, white collar, everybody.
> It's nonstop. It's every day. And
> it doesn't seem like it's getting
> any better."
>
> —Walter Bender, deputy
> sheriff of Montgomery
> County, Ohio

Statistics regarding the opioid crisis paint a sobering picture. On average, drug overdoses kill more than 64,000 people in the United States every year, and they have dragged down the country's average life expectancy by at least two years.[1] In 2019, opioid overdoses were responsible for 70.6 percent of all overdose deaths.[2] Since the beginning of the COVID-19 pandemic in early 2020, the opioid crisis has only gotten deadlier. According to data from the Centers for Disease Control and Prevention (CDC)'s National Center for Health Statistics, between April 2020 and April 2021 there were approximately 75,673 overdose deaths from opioids, driving the annual overdose rate for all drugs to above 100,000.[3] Since 1990, opioid overdoses have accounted for over 600,000 deaths in the U.S. and Canada, which exceeds the total American fatalities in World War I and World War II combined.[4] Though incomparable to the human loss of the opioid crisis, its financial impact is also devastating. A 2022 bipartisan report from the U.S. Congress estimates that drug overdoses cost the country approximately $1 trillion every year due to the premature deaths of workers, criminal justice costs, and health-care costs.[5]

It may seem surprising that this could be allowed to happen in a country as privileged as the United States, but the circumstances surrounding the beginning of today's opioid crisis shed light on this situation. In 1996, the American pharmaceutical company Purdue Pharma introduced the drug OxyContin, a prescription opioid that is intended to relieve severe pain.[6] The aggressive marketing of OxyContin to physicians, combined with Purdue Pharma's deceptive misrepresentation of the risk of addiction to the drug, resulted in many patients becoming inadvertently addicted to opioids. According to a report by the U.S. Department of Justice, Purdue Pharma officials were aware that OxyContin was being abused the same year that it was released, but they concealed this information and continued to market the drug as being less prone to addiction and abuse than other prescription opioids.[7]

Chronic pain is a serious issue in the United States: according to the CDC, 20.4 percent of American adults suffered from chronic pain in 2019.[8] Prescription opioids seemed like a great solution to this problem, since they were specifically marketed as a treatment for chronic pain. However, this treatment often came at a deadly cost. Between 1999 and 2006, the prescription opioid death rate continued to rise. But starting in 2007 the death rate started to slow due to awareness in the medical community of the addictiveness of prescription opioids—which in turn led to changes in prescription practices—and legal action against pharmaceutical companies.[9] The hope was that the decrease in prescriptions would lead to decreased opioid addiction and overdose deaths, but unfortunately this only led to an even deadlier stage of the opioid crisis.

Once prescription opioids became more difficult to obtain, many people who had become addicted to opioids turned to illegal opioids instead. Initially the replacement drug of choice was heroin. The availability and low price of heroin made it an attractive alternative to people who had developed addictions to prescription opioids, and research indicates that people who previously used prescription opioids are 13 times as likely to start using heroin compared to people who have never used opioids.[10] Despite the relatively low price of heroin, fentanyl was even cheaper, and around 2013 heroin dealers started to cut their product with fentanyl.[11] Fentanyl is a synthetic opioid that is used as a medication for severe pain. Often, people who consume the drug illegally do not knowingly do so, since dealers mix it with other drugs to increase the potency and cut down on the cost. Fentanyl is considerably more potent and deadlier than heroin, and its increased use caused fentanyl overdose deaths to climb by 88 percent per year between 2013 and 2016.[12]

The opioid crisis in the United States has devastated countless communities, families, and individuals. It has dragged down the nation's life expectancy and economy, and it has not just persisted but grown over the decades since it started. Policymakers, healthcare professionals, law enforcement, and concerned citizens have tried to make sense of what is responsible for this devastating addiction crisis, which populations are most vulnerable to its impacts, and how the opioid crisis can finally be stopped. In chapters titled "What Caused the Opioid Crisis?"; "What Are the Demographics of the Opioid Crisis?"; "Who Is Responsible for the Opioid Crisis, and Can They Be Held Accountable?"; and "Can the Opioid Crisis Be Stopped?", the viewpoints in *Opposing Viewpoints: The Opioid Crisis* examine a wide range of perspectives from experts on these topics in an effort to help make sense of this grave threat to American society.

Notes

1. James Nachtwey, "The Opioid Diaries," *TIME*, 2018. https://time.com/james-nachtwey-opioid-addiction-america/.
2. "Maps and Graphs on U.S. Drug Overdose Death Rates," U.S. Centers for Disease Control and Prevention (CDC), February 22, 2022. https://www.cdc.gov/drugoverdose/deaths/index.html.
3. National Center for Health Statistics, "Drug Overdose Deaths in the U.S. Top 100,000," U.S. Centers for Disease Control and Prevention (CDC), November 17, 2021. https://www.cdc.gov/nchs/pressroom/nchs_press_releases/2021/20211117.htm.
4. Robert Hart, "1.2 Million Opioid Overdose Deaths Expected in U.S. and Canada by 2029, Experts Warn," *Forbes*, February 2, 2022. https://www.forbes.com/sites/roberthart/2022/02/02/12-million-opioid-overdose-deaths-expected-in-us-and-canada-by-2029-experts-warn/?sh=48de33723da3.

5. Chloe Taylor, "Drug overdoses are costing the U.S. economy $1 trillion a year, government report estimates," *CNBC*, February 8, 2022. https://www.cnbc.com/2022/02/08/drug-overdoses-cost-the-us-around-1-trillion-a-year-report-says.html.

6. Art Van Zee, "The Promotion and Marketing of OxyContin: Commercial Triumph, Public Health Tragedy," *American Journal of Public Health*, February 2009. https://www.ncbi.nlm.nih.gov/pmc/articles/PMC2622774/.

7. Barry Meier, "Origins of an Epidemic: Purdue Pharma Knew Its Opioids Were Widely Abused," *New York Times*, May 29, 2018. https://www.nytimes.com/2018/05/29/health/purdue-opioids-oxycontin.html.

8. Carla E. Zelaya et al., "Chronic Pain and High-Impact Chronic Pain Among U.S. Adults, 2019," National Center for Health Statistics, November 2020. https://www.cdc.gov/nchs/products/databriefs/db390.htm.

9. Steve Sternberg and Gaby Galvin, "America's Deadly New Normal," *US News & World Report,* January 28, 2019. https://www.usnews.com/news/health-news/articles/2019-01-28/opioid-crisis-points-to-deadly-new-normal-for-america.

10. Magdalena Cerdá et al., "Nonmedical Prescription Opioid Use in Childhood and Early Adolescence Predicts Transitions to Heroin Use in Young Adulthood: A National Study," *Journal of Pediatrics,* September 2015. https://pubmed.ncbi.nlm.nih.gov/26054942/.

11. Sarah DeWeerdt, "Tracing the US Opioid Crisis to Its Roots," *Nature,* September 11, 2019. https://www.nature.com/articles/d41586-019-02686-2.

12. *Ibid.*

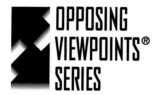

CHAPTER 1

What Caused the Opioid Crisis?

Chapter Preface

W hat is responsible for the massive scale of human loss caused by the opioid crisis, and why did this crisis explode in the 1990s? Opium—which is a naturally produced type of opioid that is made from the sap of the opium poppy—has been used medicinally and recreationally for thousands of years.[1] Its first recorded use was in ancient Mesopotamia in around the year 3,400 BCE, and subsequent records indicate that it was also used in ancient Greece, Persia, and Egypt.[2] Modern opioid use can be traced back to the early 1800s, when morphine was first extracted from opium by the German pharmacist Friedrich Serturner.[3] Morphine is a very powerful painkiller, and it is also highly addictive. It was widely used in the United States to address a range of ailments in the nineteenth century, but use of morphine took off exponentially during the U.S. Civil War (1861–1865) to treat soldiers wounded in battle.[4] By 1895, approximately 1 in 200 Americans were addicted to opium powder or morphine.[5] As a response to the alarming addiction rates, the Harrison Narcotic Act of 1914 was passed to significantly limit the distribution and use of opiates in both medical and recreational settings.[6]

Even though the opioid crisis following the U.S. Civil War demonstrated what a destructive and widespread impact opioid addiction could have, history repeated itself at the turn of the twenty-first century, leading to even more devastation than the previous crisis. Purdue Pharma is frequently blamed for starting today's opioid crisis, as their marketing strategies encouraged doctors to prescribe the opioid OxyContin, resulting in the use of opioids by millions of patients. Even more problematic is the fact that the company's deceptive practices caused doctors to be misinformed about the effects of the drug, including its addictiveness. Purdue Pharma claimed that the drug would provide pain relief to patients for twelve hours, making it a longer-lasting pain control option than other drugs on the market and allowing patients to take fewer pills. However, this proved to be untrue. Records indicate that the effects of the drug wear off after fewer than 12 hours and that patients experience withdrawals between the two pills, causing them to develop a craving that nurtured addiction.[7] What's more, records suggest that Purdue Pharma officials were aware of this, as well as the fact that the drug was frequently being abused.[8]

Once an addiction to opioids develops, it is extremely difficult to kick. This is because of the effects opioids have on the brain. Opioids cause those who use them to develop a strong dependency because they impair the brain's decision-making abilities and take over its reward center, causing an opioid user to crave and seek more opioids without regard for the negative effects this may have.[9] By the time regulation of prescription opioids tightened and they became more difficult to obtain, many opioid users were already hooked. Some turned to illegal drugs that tended to be cheaper and easier to find than prescription opioids, like heroin and fentanyl, to soothe their craving. What makes opioids particularly dangerous is how deadly they are. Their effects on the respiratory system and heart cause users to be particularly susceptible to deadly overdoses.[10]

The viewpoints in this chapter consider the many variables that led to the opioid crisis and caused it to worsen. Experts discuss the biological effects of opioids, the historical context of America's opioid use, the marketing practices of pharmaceutical companies like Purdue Pharma, the socioeconomic factors that drive people to opioid use, and pharmaceutical regulation in the U.S.

Notes

1. History.com Editors, "Heroin, Morphine and Opium," History.com, June 10, 2019. https://www.history.com/topics/crime/history-of-heroin-morphine-and-opiates.
2. *Ibid.*
3. Ramtin Arablouei and Rund Abdelfatah, "A History of Opioids in America," *NPR*, April 4, 2019. https://www.npr.org/2019/04/04/709767408/a-history-of-opioids-in-america.
4. *Ibid.*

5. Erick Trickey, "Inside the Story of America's 19th-Century Opiate Addiction," *Smithsonian Magazine*, January 4, 2018. https://www.smithsonianmag.com/history/inside-story-americas-19th-century-opiate-addiction-180967673/.

6. *Ibid.*

7. Eve Cable, "How Purdue Pharma Got Away with It All," *McGill Daily*, September 20, 2021. https://www.mcgilldaily.com/2021/09/how-purdue-pharma-got-away-with-it-all/.

8. *Ibid.*

9. Lauren Gravitz, "Unravelling the Mystery of Opioid Addiction," *Nature,* September 11, 2019. https://www.nature.com/articles/d41586-019-02690-6.

10. Carrie Krieger, "What Makes Opioid Medications So Dangerous?" Mayo Clinic. https://www.mayoclinic.org/diseases-conditions/prescription-drug-abuse/expert-answers/what-are-opioids/faq-20381270.

> *"Today, doctors are re-learning lessons their predecessors learned more than a lifetime ago. Opium's history in the United States is as old as the nation itself."*

America Has a Long History of Opioid Addiction

Erick Trickey

In the following viewpoint, Erick Trickey explains that today's opioid crisis is not entirely unprecedented in U.S. history. The U.S. Civil War (1861–65) wounded hundreds of thousands of soldiers. For doctors treating these soldiers suffering from devastating injuries, morphine seemed like a wonder drug. It quickly helped relieve pain caused by a massive range of medical conditions. After the war ended, doctors continued to frequently prescribe opium powders and morphine. However, it eventually became clear that these drugs were extremely addictive, and by the early 20th century regulations were in place to control opioid use. Nonetheless, illegal opioid use persisted. Erick Trickey is a journalist who writes about history and politics.

As you read, consider the following questions:

1. According to the author, how common was opioid addiction in America by 1895?
2. What are some of the conditions listed in the viewpoint that were treated with opioids?
3. What is one law mentioned in the viewpoint that was passed to help regulate opioid use?

The man was bleeding, wounded in a bar fight, half-conscious. Charles Schuppert, a New Orleans surgeon, was summoned to help. It was the late 1870s, and Schuppert, like thousands of American doctors of his era, turned to the most effective drug in his kit. "I gave him an injection of morphine subcutaneously of ½ grain," Schuppert wrote in his casebook. "This acted like a charm, as he came to in a minute from the stupor he was in and rested very easily."

Physicians like Schuppert used morphine as a new-fangled wonder drug. Injected with a hypodermic syringe, the medication relieved pain, asthma, headaches, alcoholics' delirium tremens, gastrointestinal diseases and menstrual cramps. "Doctors were really impressed by the speedy results they got," says David T. Courtwright, author of Dark Paradise: A History of Opiate Addiction in America. "It's almost as if someone had handed them a magic wand."

By 1895, morphine and opium powders, like OxyContin and other prescription opioids today, had led to an addiction epidemic that affected roughly 1 in 200 Americans. Before 1900, the typical opiate addict in America was an upper-class or middle-class white woman. Today, doctors are re-learning lessons their predecessors learned more than a lifetime ago.

Opium's history in the United States is as old as the nation itself. During the American Revolution, the Continental and British armies used opium to treat sick and wounded soldiers. Benjamin Franklin took opium late in life to cope with severe pain from a bladder stone. A doctor gave laudanum, a tincture of opium mixed with alcohol, to Alexander Hamilton after his fatal duel with Aaron Burr.

The Civil War helped set off America's opiate epidemic. The Union Army alone issued nearly 10 million opium pills to its soldiers, plus 2.8 million ounces of opium powders and tinctures. An unknown number of soldiers returned home addicted, or with war wounds that opium relieved. "Even if a disabled soldier survived the war without becoming addicted, there was a good chance he would later meet up with a hypodermic-wielding physician," Courtright wrote. The hypodermic syringe, introduced to the United States in 1856 and widely used to deliver morphine by the 1870s, played an even greater role, argued Courtwright in Dark Paradise. "Though it could cure little, it could relieve anything," he wrote. "Doctors and patients alike were tempted to overuse."

Opiates made up 15 percent of all prescriptions dispensed in Boston in 1888, according to a survey of the city's drug stores. "In 1890, opiates were sold in an unregulated medical marketplace," wrote Caroline Jean Acker in her 2002 book, Creating the American Junkie: Addiction Research in the Classic Era of Narcotic Control. "Physicians prescribed them for a wide range of indications, and pharmacists sold them to individuals medicating themselves for physical and mental discomforts."

Male doctors turned to morphine to relieve many female patients' menstrual cramps, "diseases of a nervous character," and even morning sickness. Overuse led to addiction. By the late 1800s, women made up more than 60 percent of opium addicts. "Uterine and ovarian complications cause more ladies to fall into the [opium] habit, than all other diseases combined," wrote Dr. Frederick Heman Hubbard in his 1881 book, The Opium Habit and Alcoholism.

Throughout the 1870s and 1880s, medical journals filled with warnings about the danger of morphine addiction. But many doctors were slow to heed them, because of inadequate medical education and a shortage of other treatments. "In the 19th century, when a physician decided to recommend or prescribe an opiate for a patient, the physician did not have a lot of alternatives," said Courtwright in a recent interview. Financial pressures mattered too: demand for morphine from well-off patients, competition from other doctors and pharmacies willing to supply narcotics.

Only around 1895, at the peak of the epidemic, did doctors begin to slow and reverse the overuse of opiates. Advances in medicine and public health played a role: acceptance of the germ theory of disease, vaccines, x-rays, and the debut of new pain relievers, such as aspirin in 1899. Better sanitation meant fewer patients contracting dysentery or other gastrointestinal diseases, then turning to opiates for their constipating and pain-relieving effects.

Educating doctors was key to fighting the epidemic. Medical instructors and textbooks from the 1890s regularly delivered strong warnings against overusing opium. "By the late 19th century, [if] you pick up a medical journal about morphine addiction," says Courtwright, "you'll very commonly encounter a sentence like this: 'Doctors who resort too quickly to the needle are lazy, they're incompetent, they're poorly trained, they're behind the times.'" New regulations also helped: state laws passed between 1895 and 1915 restricted the sale of opiates to patients with a valid prescription, ending their availability as over-the-counter drugs.

As doctors led fewer patients to addiction, another kind of user emerged as the new face of the addict. Opium smoking spread across the United States from the 1870s into the 1910s, with Chinese immigrants operating opium dens in most major cities and Western towns. They attracted both indentured Chinese immigrant workers and white Americans, especially "lower-class urban males, often neophyte members of the underworld," according to Dark Paradise. "It's a poor town now-a-days that has not a Chinese laundry," a white opium-smoker said in 1883, "and nearly every one of these has its layout"—an opium pipe and accessories.

That shift created a political opening for prohibition. "In the late 19th century, as long as the most common kind of narcotic addict was a sick old lady, a morphine or opium user, people weren't really interested in throwing them in jail," Courtwright says. "That was a bad problem, that was a scandal, but it wasn't a crime."

That changed in the 1910s and 1920s, he says. "When the typical drug user was a young tough on a street corner, hanging out with his friends and snorting heroin, that's a very different and less sympathetic picture of narcotic addiction."

The federal government's efforts to ban opium grew out of its new colonialist ambitions in the Pacific. The Philippines were then a territory under American control, and the opium trade there raised significant concerns. President Theodore Roosevelt called for an international opium commission to meet in Shanghai at the urging of alarmed American missionaries stationed in the region. "U.S. delegates," wrote Acker in Creating the American Junkie, "were in a poor position to advocate reform elsewhere when their own country lack national legislation regulating the opium trade." Secretary of State Elihu Root submitted a draft bill to Congress that would ban the import of opium prepared for smoking and punish possession of it with up to two years in prison. "Since smoking opium was identified with Chinese, gamblers, and prostitutes," Courtwright wrote, "little opposition was anticipated."

The law, passed in February 1909, limited supply and drove prices up. One New York City addict interviewed for a study quoted in Acker's book said the price of "a can of hop" jumped from $4 to $50. That pushed addicts toward more potent opiates, especially morphine and heroin.

The subsequent Harrison Narcotic Act of 1914, originally intended as a regulation of medical opium, became a near-prohibition. President Woodrow Wilson's Treasury Department used the act to stamp out many doctors' practice of prescribing opiates to "maintain" an addict's habit. After the U.S. Supreme Court endorsed this interpretation of the law in 1919, cities across the nation opened narcotic clinics for the addicted—a precursor to modern methadone treatment. The clinics were short-lived; the Treasury Department's Narcotic Division succeeded in closing nearly all of them by 1921. But those that focused on long-term maintenance and older, sicker addicts—such as Dr. Willis Butler's clinic in Shreveport, Louisiana—showed good results, says Courtwright. "One of the lessons of the 20th-century treatment saga," he says, "is that long term maintenance can work, and work very well, for some patients."

Courtwright, a history professor at the University of North Florida, wrote Dark Paradise in 1982, then updated it in 2001 to include post-World War II heroin addiction and the Reagan-era war on drugs. Since then, he's been thinking a lot about the similarities and differences between America's two major opiate epidemics, 120 years apart. Modern doctors have a lot more treatment options than their 19th-century counterparts, he says, but they experienced a much more organized commercial campaign that pressed them to prescribe new opioids such as OxyContin. "The wave of medical opiate addiction in the 19th century was more accidental," says Courtwright. "In the late 20th and early 21st centuries, there's more of a sinister commercial element to it."

In 1982, Courtwright wrote, "What we think about addiction very much depends on who is addicted." That holds true today, he says. "You don't see a lot of people advocating a 1980s-style draconian drug policy with mandatory minimum sentences in response to this epidemic," he says.

Class and race play a role in that, he acknowledges. "A lot of new addicts are small-town white Americans: football players who get their knees messed up in high school or college, older people who have a variety of chronic degenerative diseases." Reversing the trend of 100 years ago, drug policy is turning less punitive as addiction spreads among middle-class, white Americans.

Now, Courtwright says, the country may be heading toward a wiser policy that blends drug interdiction with treatment and preventive education. "An effective drug policy is concerned with both supply reduction and demand reduction," he says. "If you can make it more difficult and expensive to get supply, at the same time that you make treatment on demand available to people, then that's a good strategy."

*"It is the precedent of overzealous
marketing to healthcare professionals
that really launched the opioid
epidemic in the late '90s and early
2000s."*

The Modern Pharmaceutical Industry Caused the Opioid Crisis

Eve Cable

Though drug addiction has been an issue in America for centuries, some of the characteristics of today's pharmaceutical industry help explain why the current opioid crisis is worse than any previous addiction crisis. In this viewpoint, Eve Cable examines how one pharmaceutical company in particular—Purdue Pharma—used advertising and marketing to healthcare professionals to sell massive amounts of opioids and ultimately fuel the opioid crisis. The author examines a number of the manipulative marketing strategies used by the company to persuade and mislead healthcare professionals. Eve Cable was a student at McGill University, where she was an editor for the McGill Daily.

As you read, consider the following questions:

1. What family owns the Purdue Pharma
    pharmaceutical company?

"How Purdue Pharma Got Away with it All," by Eve Cable, The McGill Daily, September 20, 2021. Reprinted by permission.

2. At the time this article was published, how many American states had sued Purdue Pharma?

3. How much did Purdue Pharma pay in bonuses to pharmaceutical sales reps in the year 2001?

P urdue Pharma began production of OxyContin—the largest contributor to opioid addiction globally—in 1995, pushing the use of the drug for a wider range of ailments than ever before as pain relief medication. Executives at Purdue Pharma continued to assert throughout the years that OxyContin led to addiction in fewer than one percent of patients, increasing widespread willingness to prescribe the drug and assuaging previous concerns concerning addictive pain medication. Most importantly, Purdue Pharma enacted one of the most relentless marketing campaigns for an opioid drug ever, essentially manipulating healthcare professionals into over-prescribing the medication, and misleading both healthcare professionals and the general public about the true nature of the drug. Since then, over 3,000 cases have been brought against Purdue Pharma from public and private claimants, with over 47 American states suing the company, 29 of which specifically name the Sackler family as defendants.

While the opioid epidemic continues to ravage communities, the Sackler family remains one of the richest families in the world, with a September 1 bankruptcy settlement absolving them from any long-term blame or accountability for their role in the crisis. The settlement, approved by federal Judge Robert Drain, grants immunity to the Sackler family in any future opioid-related lawsuits, while simultaneously marketing meagre payouts for those affected as a "solution" to the years of pain and suffering the family has caused. While it may seem as though one of America's richest families has narrowly avoided prosecution, the Sacklers have spent more than a quarter of a century profiting from opioid addiction and deaths— all while keeping themselves at an arm's length from legal matters concerning the drug and Purdue Pharma. At the end of it all, the

Sacklers will still remain one of America's wealthiest families. This begs the question: how did they manage that?

It is crucial to note that the Sackler family's ability to absolve themselves of any blame and responsibility in the opioid crisis is not a last-minute stroke of luck. Rather, it is the success of years of calculated manoeuvres that set the family up for long-term financial security and minimal legal accountability. The three most central figures in the family are Arthur, Mortimer and Raymond Sackler, who bought pharmaceutical company Purdue-Frederick in 1952. While Mortimer and Raymond took responsibility for Purdue itself, Arthur became the biggest name in the new field of medical advertising. This connection would be a key foundation for the massive amounts of marketing that Purdue Pharma would go on to do for OxyContin. While Arthur Sackler died in 1987 and OxyContin production did not start until 1995, his widow Jillian's claims that he should be removed from any discussion of the opioid crisis are purposely ignorant of his contributions to Purdue's investment in medical advertising. "Where his brothers built their reputation manufacturing and selling pharmaceuticals, Arthur Sackler gained his business renown by promoting them," Christopher Rowland writes in The Washington Post.

While the opioid epidemic continues to ravage communities, the Sackler family remains one of richest families in the world.

This is the cornerstone of Purdue Pharma's identity: relentless advertising and marketing to healthcare professionals. Arthur Sackler helped build that identity by becoming a leading expert in the field of medical advertising, while Raymond and Mortimer Sackler used their clinical expertise alongside this foundation to launch OxyContin into the big leagues of prescription pain medication. Though Arthur died before the release of the drug itself, he was no doubt a key contributor to the corporate culture of malicious over-advertising for profit. Jillian Sackler's desire to protect her late husband's name is a subtle yet downright offensive way of overwriting the ways in which the Sackler family has organized to protect their financial interests from the very beginning of their business ventures.

It is the precedent of overzealous marketing to healthcare professionals that really launched the opioid epidemic in the late '90s and early 2000s. Between 1996 and 2001, Purdue hosted over 5,000 pharmacists, physicians and nurses in attractive, all-expenses-paid symposiums, where healthcare professionals were trained liberally in the benefits of prescribing OxyContin. These symposiums, held often in "popular sunbelt vacation sites," played an active role in healthcare professionals' willingness to over prescribe medication. While most clinicians who attended these symposiums believed that enticing trips "would not alter their prescribing patterns," researchers Orlowski and Wateska have compiled data to prove the contrary, arguing that attending events such as these leads to "a significant increase in the prescribing patterns" of the drugs being discussed during the conference.

Another incredibly sinister aspect of Purdue Pharma's marketing scheme regarding OxyContin was its abuse of data from physicians around the US in order to concretely target certain communities. Using physician data, executives were able to identify which doctors prescribed the most opioids, then target those clinicians with more advertising. While Purdue Pharma and Sackler family members claim this was to identify "physicians with large numbers of chronic pain patients," the database also identifies "which physicians were simply the most frequent prescribers of opioids and, in some cases, the least discriminate prescribers." Ultimately, Purdue weaponised large amounts of physical health data to maximise their sales reach, with no real regard for the patients at the centre of it all.

The other factors that increased OxyContin sales in terms of marketing were a "lucrative bonus system" for sales representatives, a patient coupon program for a free month-long prescription of the medication, and the distribution of promotional items. While the average sales representative's salary for the company in 2001 was US $55,000, Purdue was paying out an average bonus of $71,500, with a cumulative $40 million paid out in bonuses to sales reps in that year alone, blatantly displaying the company's impetus to keep their sales reps selling vast quantities of OxyContin. The message that OxyContin had a "less than one per cent risk of addiction," a statistic based on studies that have since been disputed, was disseminated across the country through sales representatives. The coupon program allowed for patients to receive a free prescription of OxyContin for a full month, and when the program was ended in 2001, over 34,000 coupons had been redeemed. While it's not uncommon for pharmaceutical companies to send branded merchandise to doctors, a plethora of stuffed toys, CDs, and clothing hit medical professionals desks, an "unprecedented" level of merchandising for such a medication, according to the Drug Enforcement Administration.

This is nothing short of conscious manipulation of medical professionals for profit, and there is a strong case that Purdue Pharma, and specifically members of the Sackler family, knew the drug to be significantly more addictive and risky than described in their advertising. This level of marketing and manipulation could only happen because of years of medical advertising expertise that was built into the fabric of the company—the groundwork laid by Arthur Sackler serving as the foundation of Purdue's calculated strategy.

Part of this strategy had to include addressing doctors' fears concerning opioid prescription, which they had long been told was high-risk and should generally be reserved for end-of-life care. Purdue's argument was that OxyContin was a different type of medicine than the drugs they had come across before, because it was a sustained-release opioid, in contrast to opiates like morphine, which are immediate-release. The protective coating on OxyContin means that the drug is slowly released into the patient's system over an extended period of 12 hours. Purdue claimed that this difference reduced the addictive nature of the drug, and made it safer for more widespread consumption than immediate release drugs like morphine. Moreover, they sought to address the issue of ongoing chronic pain, and argued that sustained-release

OxyContin was better for managing constant or ongoing pain than immediate-release options. However, the FDA's medical review officer in 1995 observed that OxyContin did not have a significant benefit for patients, and that similar results were achieved with immediate-release oxycodone.

Purdue Pharma made OxyContin seem like a lifeline for sufferers of chronic pain. A drug that would allow relief for 12 full hours, longer than most other competitors, and only two pills to take per day, which would provide, according to Purdue, "smooth and sustained pain control all day and all night." With Purdue Pharma continually claiming that the drug carried only a one per cent risk of addiction, it seemed like a medical miracle for individuals who had previously found no solutions for their pain conditions.

However, for most patients, internal Purdue documents have shown that the drug, for many people, did not offer 12 hour relief. Instead, individuals began to experience withdrawals during the interim period between pills, experiencing "body aches, nausea, anxiety and other symptoms of withdrawal." This suggests that the higher dose extended release pill was releasing the dose quicker than desired, essentially rendering the "extended release" function of the drug useless and sending patients into withdrawal. An LA Times investigation into this 12 hour problem noted that "when the agony is relieved by the next dose, it creates a cycle of pain and euphoria that fosters addiction."

This is nothing short of conscious manipulation of medical professionals for profit, and there is a strong case that Purdue Pharma […] knew the drug to be significantly more addictive and risky than described in their advertising.

Purdue had created the perfect storm for an epidemic of addiction, and their executives, including members of the Sackler family, have been quick to deny any intent in this respect, claiming that they had no role to play in the opioid epidemic and that their genuine goal was to relieve pain. However, internal documents prove that to be false—in fact, OxyContin was made to replace a previous Purdue product called MS Contin, which was no longer a moneymaker for the company. In a 1990 memo, Purdue scientist Robert Kaiko made it clear that the expiration of MS Contin's patent would lead to a decrease in revenue for the company: "MS Contin may eventually face serious generic competition." Therefore, the company was determined to find a new cash flow, but they needed it to stand out from pain medications that other pharmaceutical companies would be releasing—it needed to be different enough from MS Contin that it was considered a brand new "miracle" drug.

Instead of demonstrating any care for sufferers of chronic pain, Purdue Pharma was entirely finance and profit-oriented. Chief executive Michael Friedman addressed Kaiko's concerns: "OxyContin can cure the vulnerability of the […] generic threat and that is why it is so crucial that we devote our fullest efforts now to a successful launch of OxyContin." Executive meetings were therefore focused on finding a "cure" to the financial threat of Big Pharma competition, not on finding a cure to patients' chronic pain.

In addition to being purely financially motivated, Purdue Pharma has also been consistently vague about what they did and did not know about OxyContin in the first months and years after the drug's release. The first trials of OxyContin were in women recovering from surgery in two Puerto Rican hospitals in 1989; these women complained of pain increase in the first eight hours, with half needing more medication before the 12 hour mark. After this clearly inconclusive study, OxyContin was somehow deemed safe, and the drug was approved as a longer-lasting painkiller despite the fact that it had failed to control patients' pain for the marketed 12 hours.

Moreover, Purdue Pharma knew years before any legal cases that addiction was an issue with their medication, and that they were contributing to widespread abuse of opioids. While the company and many individual Sackler family members have claimed that they knew only years after OxyContin's release that it was dangerous, internal files from 1996 reveal a different story. Executives knew that pills were being crushed and snorted, with the company's sales reps using the words "street value," "crush" and "snort" in

117 notes from visits to medical professionals between 1997 and 1999. The crushing of pills removes the protective film that makes the medication extended release, therefore meaning that individuals were receiving an extremely high dose of medication directly into their bloodstream. Purdue Pharma's sales representatives clearly acknowledged there was evidence of OxyContin being crushed and snorted; executives' failure to intervene despite this knowledge leaves the blood of millions on their hands.

Purdue Pharma knew years before any legal cases that addiction was an issue with their medication, and that they were contributing to widespread abuse of opioids.

Purdue Pharma and members of the Sackler family knew what their drug was doing to people sooner than they claimed. The evidence for this is objective, written in internal memos and shared multiple times in court depositions, both in the 2007 case against the company and in the bankruptcy case this year. To see the Sackler family walk away with immunity from all future opioid related lawsuits is evidence of both the court and country's lack of care for the victims of addiction, and demonstrates an obsession with pandering to the needs of the wealthiest corporations and members of society.

Bankruptcy court was the Sacklers' way out of the OxyContin crisis, but for hundreds of thousands of individuals and families across America and the world, the crisis leaves permanent irreparable damage to their lives and communities, including the loss of at least 500,000 lives. While the Sacklers made an absolute minimum of $10 billion from the sales of OxyContin, the thousands of people whose lives have been ravaged by the opioid crisis will be unable to sue the Sacklers for the damage done, essentially the last nail in the coffin for seeking any small form of justice. Purdue Pharma and the Sackler family are responsible for what New York's attorney general, Letitia James, describes as "the taproot of the opioid epidemic;" they have blood on their hands, and they're getting away with it.

> *"Understanding deaths of despair extends not just to pinpointing the relative importance of drug supply and demand factors, but also to what 'despair' means."*

Economic Despair in the U.S. Led to Increased Opioid Addiction and Overdose Deaths

Clark Merrefield

In the following viewpoint, Clark Merrefield examines recent research on the connection between economic despair and the rise in opioid drug overdoses, which are often categorized as "deaths of despair." Job opportunities—especially well-paying ones— have decreased for people without a college education. This has particularly impacted working class white populations in economically depressed parts of the country. However, Black, Latinx, and American Indian populations have also experienced increased rates of deaths of despair. The growing sense of hopelessness combined with the greater supply of opioids—first prescription opioids, then illegal drugs—was a recipe for disaster. Clark Merrefield is a reporter at the Journalist's Resource.

As you read, consider the following questions:

1. According to this viewpoint, how many drug overdose deaths occurred in the U.S. between April 2020 and April 2021?
2. What does the author consider to be "deaths of despair" in this viewpoint?
3. Which five states required doctors to fill out three copies of prescriptions in 1996, when the drug OxyContin was introduced?

L ate last year, the National Center for Health Statistics released provisional data showing a large increase in drug overdose deaths from April 2020 to April 2021.

The center estimates 100,306 drug overdose deaths in the U.S. over that time, a 29% rise from 78,056 overdose deaths over the same period one year prior.

Drug overdose deaths are one part of what Princeton University economists Anne Case and Angus Deaton term "deaths of despair." Liver disease from alcohol use and suicide are the other contributors.

Case and Deaton first described the contours of deaths of despair in the U.S. in an influential 2015 paper and a follow-up paper in 2017. Their fundamental assertion is the rise in deaths from drugs, alcohol and self-harm was spurred by decades of decline in economic opportunity for middle-aged people with relatively low levels of education.

The bulk of those additional 20,000-plus deaths during the first throes of the COVID-19 pandemic were related to overdoses of fentanyl, the synthetic opioid 50 to 100 times more potent than morphine, according to the data. The figures include accidental and intentional overdoses.

"Many of these deaths also involved other drugs, such as methamphetamine and cocaine, with which fentanyl-related substances may be mixed—often without the knowledge of the people who take them," Nora Volkow, director of the

National Institute on Drug Abuse, testified during a December 2021 Congressional hearing.

Total deaths from cirrhosis and other liver ailments caused by alcohol use have steadily risen since the late 1990s, peaking at 29,505 in 2020, the most recent year available. The death rate from liver disease related to heavy drinking reached 9 per 100,000 people in 2020, up from 4.3 per 100,000 in 1999.

Suicide has likewise trended upward over the past two decades, but fell from a high of 48,312 deaths in 2018 to 45,940 last year. The suicide rate remained elevated in 2020 at 13.9 per 100,000 people, up from 10.5 per 100,000 in 1999.

"The increase in deaths of despair was almost all among those without a bachelor's degree," Case and Deaton write in their March 2020 book on the topic. "Those with a four-year degree are mostly exempt; it is those without the degree who are at risk."

For some population subgroups, the rise of deaths of despair in the U.S. has been substantial, even before the pandemic. In their 2017 paper, "Mortality and Morbidity in the 21st Century," Case and Deaton note the mortality rate for white people aged 50 to 54 with only a high school diploma was nearly one-third lower in 1999 than for Black people in the same age group with any level of education.

By 2015, the situation had flipped: using the same categories, the mortality rate was nearly one-third higher for white people than for Black people.

"Ultimately, we see our story as about the collapse of the white working class after its heyday in the early 1970s, and the pathologies that accompany that decline," they write.

Recent Research Suggests Deaths of Despair Not Exclusively a White, Working Class Problem

Subsequent research from Case and Deaton and others suggests deaths of despair are not exclusively a white, working-class problem. Steven Woolf, a professor of family medicine and population health at Virginia Commonwealth University, and Heidi Schoomaker, a

The Benefits and Dangers of Opioids

When used as directed by your doctor, opioid medications safely help control acute pain, such as pain you experience after surgery. There are risks, though, when the medications are used incorrectly.

What Opioid Medications Do

Opioids are a broad group of pain-relieving drugs that work by interacting with opioid receptors in your cells. Opioids can be made from the poppy plant—for example, morphine (Kadian, MS Contin, others)—or synthesized in a laboratory—for example, fentanyl (Actiq, Duragesic, others).

When opioid medications travel through your blood and attach to opioid receptors in your brain cells, the cells release signals that muffle your perception of pain and boost your feelings of pleasure.

When Opioid Medications Are Dangerous

What makes opioid medications effective for treating pain can also make them dangerous.

At lower doses, opioids may make you feel sleepy, but higher doses can slow your breathing and heart rate, which can lead to death. And the feelings of pleasure that result from taking an opioid can make you want to continue experiencing those feelings, which may lead to addiction.

You can reduce your risk of dangerous side effects by following your doctor's instructions carefully and taking your medication exactly as prescribed. Make sure your doctor knows all of the other medications and supplements you're taking.

"What Are Opioids and Why Are They Dangerous?" by Carrie Krieger, Mayo Clinic.

student at Eastern Virginia Medical School, Norfolk, explore the geographic and racial contours of deaths of despair in a November 2019 paper in the Journal of the American Medical Association, building on a 2018 paper by Woolf and others.

Woolf and Schoomaker find, for example, that from 1999 to 2017, rural, white populations in the U.S. experienced an increase in midlife drug overdose deaths of 749%—from 4 deaths per 100,000 people to nearly 34 deaths per 100,000. But midlife drug overdose deaths rose sharply for white people living in metropolitan counties, too—a 531% increase over the same period. The drug overdose death rate among that group moved from 6.7 deaths per 100,000 to 42.5 deaths per 100,000.

The highest increase in drug overdose deaths for middle-aged white people happened in the suburbs of cities with more than 1 million residents. In those suburbs, the overdose death rate for midlife white people jumped 858%, from 4.7 deaths per 100,000 to 45.2 deaths per 100,000. Midlife drug overdose death rates for Hispanic people also peaked highest in the suburbs of large cities, according to the paper.

For Black people, the overdose death rate increased the most in cities with less than 250,000 people—but among Black people aged 55 to 64, those living in large cities experienced the biggest increase. Suicides were up the most for Black and white adults in rural counties. For Hispanic people and American Indians, suicides rose the most in metropolitan areas.

"The causes of economic despair may be more nuanced; perceptions and frustrated expectations may matter as much as absolute income or net worth," Woolf and Schoomaker write in their 2019 paper. The rate of increase of deaths of despair, they note, was generally lower on the coasts and in states with strong economic growth, such as Texas.

The crumbling economic conditions that Case and Deaton point to, particularly the declining availability of well-paying jobs for people without a college degree, fall under what economists call demand-side factors. The idea is that despair stemming from a lack of good jobs has led people to demand drugs and alcohol, and has led to self-harm.

As economists, Case and Deaton naturally focus on the financial difficulties individuals and families face. But in their 2020 book and academic writings, they also explore myriad social changes that come into play. As they put it in their book, "we see the decline in wages as slowly undermining all aspects of people's lives."

Wages adjusted for inflation have lost ground for white men without a college degree since 1979, according to Case and Deaton. Plus, "the wage decline has come with job decline—from better jobs to worse jobs—with many leaving the labor force altogether because the worse jobs are unattractive, because there are few jobs at all, or because they cannot easily move, or some combination of these reasons," they write.

The supply-side narrative centers on the supply of opioids rising in the U.S. at the stroke of a doctor's pen. With more opioids available, more people were exposed to them, meaning more people became addicted. Journalists have covered the supply side angle in books and articles, but it's less explored in academic research.

"Although there is general agreement that the causes of the crisis include a combination of supply- and demand-side factors, and interactions between them, there is less consensus regarding the relative importance of each," writes Temple University health and labor economist Catherine Maclean and co-authors in a National Bureau of Economic Research working paper published November 2020.

Case and Deaton, in their own National Bureau of Economic Research working paper from September 2021, offer that demand for opioids came first. "Pain and despair created a baseline demand for opioids, but the escalation of addiction came from pharma and its political enablers," they write.

That's not to say there is no supply-side research.

Marketing an Opioid Crisis

The rise of drug overdoses in the U.S. is, in part, a story of marketing. Marketing is the process by which a company connects a product to a market. A market is a group of people who want—or need—to buy a product.

Successful marketing is achieved through the act of selling. Selling is about convincing consumers that a product is worth their money. The proposition becomes more of a slam dunk if someone else, such as a health insurance company, is paying for it. Selling is yet more effective if trusted messengers, such as doctors, vouch for the product.

Here, the drug is oxycodone. The product is OxyContin. The company is Purdue Frederick.

OxyContin hit the pain medication market in 1996, with promotion and sales "managed by the company's marketing arm, Purdue Pharma, launched in the nation's best-known corporate tax haven—Delaware," writes journalist Beth Macy in her 2018 book, Dopesick: Dealers, Doctors and the Drug Company that Addicted America. "Purdue Pharma touted the safety of its new opioid-delivery system everywhere its merchants went."

One recent academic paper is among the first to use real-world evidence to explore supply factors that have fueled the opioid crisis. The August 2021 research in the Quarterly Journal of Economics finely traces how Purdue Pharma marketed OxyContin to American doctors and patients for decades, and how three pieces of paper saved parts of the country from being quite so hard hit by opioids.

When Purdue Pharma introduced OxyContin in the mid-1990s, there were five states requiring that every prescription have three copies. The prescribing doctor kept one copy, the pharmacy kept another and sent the third to a state drug-monitoring program.

Prescriptions, in other words, had to be filled out in triplicate.

California, Idaho, Illinois, New York, and Texas were triplicate states in 1996, accounting for roughly one-third of the nation's adult population at the time. The Department of Justice classifies oxycodone as a schedule II drug, meaning it has a "high potential for abuse which may lead to severe psychological or physical dependence."

"An earlier line of academic research found these triplicate programs had a really chilling effect in the prescribing of these schedule II drugs," says Abby Alpert, one of the paper's authors and an assistant professor of health care management at the University of Pennsylvania. "That suggested, first of all, doctors didn't want their prescribing monitored by the government. And it was also just an additional hassle for doctors."

Purdue Pharma took notice as it conducted research into marketing OxyContin as a viable pain management option for patients without cancer. Oxycodone would be delivered via a time-released pill, with the drug entering the bloodstream over 12 hours.

"Unless there is hard data to suggest otherwise, we do not feel that any further research of OxyContin for non-cancer pain would be appropriate in the triplicate states," company representatives concluded following a focus group with doctors held prior to launch, according to a batch of documents Alpert and her co-authors obtained using open records requests to the U.S. Drug Enforcement Agency. "In our judgment, the data from Texas seems to be very convincing relative to the attitudes of 'triplicate' doctors toward Class II narcotics, and unless there is reason to believe this could be different in another market (i.e., California, New York) than [sic] the findings from the Houston groups should be considered valid for all markets."

Yearly overdose death rates were slightly higher in triplicate states in the decade before OxyContin's 1996 arrival, "but this flips within a few years of the launch," Alpert and her co-authors write in the paper, "Origins of the Opioid Crisis and its Enduring Impacts."

While the drug overdose death rate rose in all states from 1996 to 2005 compared with the prior decade, the increase was relatively limited in triplicate states. By 2000, OxyContin distribution per person was 2.5 times higher in states without the triplicate prescription program compared with triplicate states.

"These large and statistically significant differences [in OxyContin distribution] persist through 2016," the authors write, even though triplicate programs had folded in the five states by 2004. If the states without a triplicate program had had a triplicate program, they would have experienced 34% fewer drug overdose deaths and 45% fewer opioid overdose deaths from 1996 to 2017, the authors estimate.

Regulatory Failures and the Need for an "Enormous Investment" in Treatment

Pain management is a real concern for doctors, particularly specialists who treat cancer and chronic conditions. OxyContin, however, was heavily marketed to primary care physicians, "who may not have been adequately trained in pain management," according to a 2003 report from the federal Government Accountability Office.

Purdue Pharma spent $700,000 on OxyContin advertising in 1996, according to the report. Purdue's strategy, along with other companies selling similar drugs, included advertising in medical journals. By 2001, Purdue's OxyContin advertising budget reached $4.1 million and OxyContin sales topped $1 billion, making it the "most frequently prescribed brand-name narcotic medication for treating moderate-to-severe pain in the United States," according to the government report.

Around the same time, news outlets began reporting on OxyContin misuse, including people crushing tablets and snorting the powder to get an immediate high, bypassing the controlled release. By the time Purdue in 2010 introduced a new OxyContin formula, which prevented rapid release of the drug when crushed, it was too late. Many of those addicted "substituted from OxyContin to heroin," Alpert and her co-authors write.

Over the years, members of the Sackler family, which bought Purdue Frederick in 1952, directed the company to market to doctors who prescribed OxyContin at high rates, "ignored and worked around safeguards intended to reduce prescription opioid misuse, and promoted false narratives about their products to steer patients away from safer alternatives and deflect blame toward people struggling with addiction," U.S. Rep. Carolyn Maloney said during a Dec. 2020 Congressional hearing.

"This is not just the fact that Purdue Pharma was marketing using false claims but also the aggressiveness and amount of advertising that also could have been maybe monitored or regulated more extensively," Alpert says.

Food and Drug Administration regulatory failures occurred from the start, according to an August 2020 commentary in the American Medical Association Journal of Ethics by Andrew Kolodny, medical director of opioid policy research at Brandeis University.

President Franklin Roosevelt signed the Food, Drug and Cosmetic Act in 1938, strengthening the government's ability to regulate the contents of food, cosmetics and drugs and barring companies from making false claims about drugs.

If the Food and Drug Administration had enforced the law, it would have labelled oxycodone only for specific, very painful conditions, according to Kolodny. The initial OxyContin label instead "featured a broad indication, allowing Purdue to promote the drug's use for common conditions for which opioids are more likely to harm than help, such as low-back pain and fibromyalgia," he writes.

Kolodny adds that while fewer doctors today are prescribing opioids, "overprescribing is still a problem. According to a recently published report, more than 2.9 million people initiated opioid use in December 2017. The FDA's continued approval of new opioids exacerbates this problem."

As Alpert notes, the U.S. is well beyond the brink of reversing the opioid crisis. "Really, now, the solution is an enormous investment in substance abuse treatment," she says.

Schoomaker, now a third-year medical student treating patients in the Norfolk, Virginia area, recalls working in an emergency department in a rural part of the state and seeing opioid overdose cases nearly every shift. In Norfolk, she has quickly observed a truism of medical treatment in the U.S.: Many patients may not see a doctor until their condition has substantially progressed. In that sense, the medical system is downstream from the economic and social factors that affect health. One way to help reduce deaths of despair could involve moving the role of the medical practitioner further upstream, Schoomaker says. It's not an easy proposition, she acknowledges, nor is it likely to be one-size-fits all.

"Those I have talked to who have much more experience say that education is really one of the key places we can be working with our patients, in describing better what their disease is, helping those folks to make informed decisions with their care and spending the time to do that," Schoomaker says. "But that's a challenge when you have 20 minutes to see a patient with a million chronic diseases—and you have a waiting room of several other patients who need to be seen that day."

Research: Raising the Wage Floor Could Reduce Deaths of Despair

There is a small but promising line of emerging research on how economic policy could reduce deaths of despair, specifically deaths stemming from intentional self-harm not involving drugs.

Research in the September 2020 issue of the Journal of Health Economics links a 10% increase in a state's minimum wage to 2.7% fewer suicides among adults with a high school diploma or less. The same increase in federal tax credits for low-income earners yields a 3% reduction in suicides among adults with less education. Those credits can vary substantially based on specific income levels and number of children.

The authors did not identify minimum wage effects on drug- and alcohol-related deaths over the period studied, 1999 to 2017, and they did not observe major suicide reductions for those with at least a bachelor's degree. The study, "Can Labor Market Policies Reduce Deaths of Despair?" covers 46 states plus Washington D.C.—the authors dropped Georgia, Oklahoma, Rhode Island and South Dakota due to incomplete data.

"Regardless of the root causes, there are some tangible policy levers we can use to try to improve population health," says Chris Lowenstein, one of the authors and a doctoral student in health policy and economics at the University of California, Berkeley.

Likewise, the authors of a January 2020 paper in the Journal of Epidemiology and Community Health look at data from all 50 states and Washington, D.C., covering 1990 to 2015, and associate a $1 minimum wage increase with a 3.4% to 5.9% decrease in the suicide rate for adults aged 18 to 64 with a high school education or less.

Deaths of despair as a concept has resonated across the media and academic landscapes. Thousands of academic papers have mentioned the phrase, according to the 2021 Case and Deaton working paper.

Understanding deaths of despair extends not just to pinpointing the relative importance of drug supply and demand factors, but also to what "despair" means.

"Despair is a concept in common use, not a well-defined diagnostic category, let alone one with a clinically validated measure," Case and Deaton write in their working paper.

National surveys on health and wellbeing do not ask about despair, per se, Case and Deaton write. Some surveys ask about pain. Case and Deaton cannot find "any study that documents falling levels of pain."

A finer understanding of how people experience despair could unlock more policy solutions.

"I think that's a good thing for people to be arguing about," Lowenstein says. "Anyone who claims to have their finger on what exactly 'despair' is, is probably going to get some pushback."

> *"When the cost … of getting painkillers rises, addicts are not dissuaded from getting their hands on these painkillers. Instead, they search for substitutes…"*

Price Theory Explains the Opiate Crisis

Zak Slayback

In the following viewpoint Zak Slayback uses basic economic concepts to illustrate how the opiate problem reached the level of crisis. He also maintains that popular policy responses are doomed to fail. Instead, pain management professionals must find alternative methods, and users must be taught to find meaning in their lives. Zak Slayback is a venture capital and private equity professional and a small business owner. He is the author of How to Get Ahead *(McGraw-Hill, 2019) and wrote the foreword to John Taylor Gatto's* Dumbing Us Down *(New Society Publishers, 2017).*

As you read, consider the following questions:

1. The author uses casualties from what war as a comparison to opiate overdoses?
2. What is inelastic demand?
3. According to the viewpoint, why does simply removing drugs from the market fail to solve the crisis?

"Price Theory Explains the Opiate Crisis," by Zak Slayback, Foundation for Economic Education, November 20, 2017. https://fee.org/articles/price-theory-explains-the-opiate-crisis/ Licensed under CC BY 4.0 International.

T he American opioid epidemic reaches new highs every year. Last year, the number of Americans killed by overdosing on opiates surpassed the number of those killed during the duration of the Vietnam War. The proliferation of fentanyl—a synthetic opiate primarily used in medical care and in tranquilizing large animals—and years upon years of medical professionals prescribing opiate painkillers for everything from a debilitating injury to a stubbed toe take the spotlight for the recent spike.

Popular policy response attacks both buckets. Against proliferation of fentanyl, considerably more dangerous and potent than heroin, some municipalities decide to charge dealers whose drugs killed users with manslaughter or even murder. Against the prescription of opiate painkillers, everybody from 60 Minutes to neighborhood moms wants it to be harder for doctors to prescribe painkillers and for it to be easier to prosecute those who recklessly do so.

This will not solve the opiate crisis. A basic exploration of economic concepts shows this.

The Economics of Addiction

The idea that most heroin and fentanyl users get started by abusing prescription painkillers is not entirely wrong. Painkillers did indeed become more common through the late 20th century and the early 21st century, peaking in 2010. The development of new drugs like OxyContin and Dilaudid and a better understanding of the anatomical features of pain in the brain gave reason for medical professionals to treat pain rather than simply trying to help clients get through it. A concentrated marketing and sales effort by pharmaceutical companies propped up by subsidies and with a long record of lobbying the government exacerbated their prescription.

This is how many opiate abusers get their start.

But how do they end up going from abusing painkillers prescribed to housewives and those with chronic pain to buying heroin and fentanyl supplied by Mexican drug cartels?

One of the first concepts taught in an ECON 101 course is that of elasticity of demand. The concept is simple. Some consumers of products show elastic demand—they will not buy (either the product or the specific brand) if the price changes even a dollar. Airline tickets are a good example of this. Most people just buy whatever the cheapest airline ticket is for their specific route, even if the slightly-more-expensive ticket may just cost a few dollars more.

Some consumers show inelastic demand—they will buy the product (or find a substitute) no matter how expensive the product gets.

The example given in nine out of ten econ courses?

Hard drug-users, like those addicted to opiates.

It's Not Enough to Remove the Drug

When the cost (including non-monetary costs like legal costs and disapprobation) of getting painkillers rises, addicts are not dissuaded from getting their hands on these painkillers. Instead, they search for substitutes—like heroin and fentanyl.

Cutting off the ability of those addicted to painkillers—whether for chronic pain or for a hedonic rush—only pushes these people from the risky-but-safer-than-heroin world of painkillers like OxyContin and Dilaudid into the blacker markets of heroin and fentanyl.

Once the addiction pathway in the brain is established, breaking that dopaminergic pathway requires building alternate pathways through deeply meaningful work and activities (this is why religious programs like 12 Step work when they do work—they help the individual tie into a deeply meaningful set of values and reward that pathway in the brain). If the pathway is merely deprived of engagement—through prohibition and then withdrawal—but not then supplemented with a pathway that overwhelms the addiction pathway, the user is just one quick decision or hit of an opiate away from falling back into the same addictive behavior.

Reducing the market in painkillers at the user-level just pushes more existing users into the black market to get their fix.

A proper response focuses on alternatives to opiate-based pain management—through less-addictive prescriptive medicine and through psychotherapy in appropriate cases—and treatment for existing addicts, not expanding prohibition.

Removing the drug from the market and from the user's body is not enough and threatens to exacerbate existing problems. Users must be able to find meaning in their lives and in their work. They must learn and be taught how to craft significant meaning for themselves and know where to find people to help them with that. They must be prepared to not merely integrate themselves back into mainstream society but go above and beyond mainstream society through seeing themselves as meaningful people through work, contribution, and education.

But that does not look good for an election campaign.

Periodical and Internet Sources Bibliography

The following articles have been selected to supplement the diverse views presented in this chapter.

Janet Currie and Hannes Schwandt, "The Opioid Epidemic Was Not Caused by Economic Distress but By Factors That Could Be More Rapidly Addressed," *Annals of the American Academy of Political and Social Science*, August 23, 2021. https://journals.sagepub.com/doi/full/10.1177/00027162211033833.

Sarah DeWeerdt, "Tracing the US Opioid Crisis to Its Roots," *Nature*, September 11, 2019. https://www.nature.com/articles/d41586-019-02686-2.

Carol Graham, "Understanding the Role of Despair in the Opioid Crisis," Brookings Institute, October 15, 2019. https://www.brookings.edu/policy2020/votervital/how-can-policy-address-the-opioid-crisis-and-despair-in-america/.

Lauren Gravitz, "Unravelling the Mystery of Opioid Addiction," *Nature,* September 11, 2019. https://www.nature.com/articles/d41586-019-02690-6.

Mark R. Jones et al., "A Brief History of the Opioid Epidemic and Strategies for Pain Management," *Pain and Therapy,* April 24, 2018. https://www.ncbi.nlm.nih.gov/pmc/articles/PMC5993682/.

Olga Khazan, "The True Cause of the Opioid Epidemic," *Atlantic*, January 2, 2020. https://www.theatlantic.com/health/archive/2020/01/what-caused-opioid-epidemic/604330/.

Catherine Maclean, Justine Mallatt, Christopher J. Ruhm, and Kosali Simon, "A Review of Economic Studies on the Opioid Crisis," *Vox EU*, December 20, 2020. https://voxeu.org/article/review-economic-studies-opioid-crisis.

Brian Mann, "More than a Million Americans Have Died from Overdoses During the Opioid Epidemic," NPR, December 30, 2021. https://www.npr.org/2021/12/30/1069062738/more-than-a-million-americans-have-died-from-overdoses-during-the-opioid-epidemi.

Barry Meier, "Origins of an Epidemic: Purdue Pharma Knew Its Opioids Were Widely Abused," *New York Times*, May 29, 2018.

https://www.nytimes.com/2018/05/29/health/purdue-opioids-oxycontin.html.

Marcia Meldrum, "Opioids' Long Shadow," *AMA Journal of Ethics,* August 2020. https://journalofethics.ama-assn.org/article/opioids-long-shadow/2020-08.

New York Times Editorial Board, "An Opioid Crisis Foretold," *New York Times*, April 21, 2018. https://www.nytimes.com/2018/04/21/opinion/an-opioid-crisis-foretold.html.

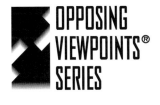

CHAPTER 2

What Are the Demographics of the Opioid Crisis?

Chapter Preface

Which groups of Americans have suffered the most harm as a result of the opioid crisis? To examine the demographics of opioid use in the U.S. is to attempt to answer this question. Demographics study patterns in society, using statistics and data to try to make sense of trends in human behavior. It is undeniable that the damage done by the opioid crisis has spread across many societal and demographic barriers, but experts have tried to examine the ways in which different characteristics could cause someone to be at greater risk of abusing or overdosing on opioids and why this may be the case. Some of the features researchers examine include gender, race, age, geographic location, education level, and socioeconomic status.

There are two variables in particular that make examining the demographics of the opioid crisis particularly challenging and cause disagreement among experts as to which groups are hit the hardest by opioid use. The first is that every person has a large number of characteristics that are used to classify them, including their age, gender, racial or ethnic background, where they live, and their financial status, among other things. To determine which of these characteristics has the greatest impact on potential opioid use involves understanding the ways these categories relate to one another.

For instance, in recent years Black Americans in urban areas have experienced rising rates of opioid overdose deaths. There are a number of potential reasons as to why this is the case, and multiple reasons could be correct. It could be because of disparities in health care related to race, which affect the type of treatment Black Americans receive for opioid addiction or whether they choose to seek treatment at all. Or it could be because unequal economic opportunities have prevented more Black Americans than white Americans from receiving quality health insurance.[1] On the flip side, these same race-based health-care disparities could have caused more white Americans to become hooked on opioids, as unequal prescription practices based on race caused more white patients to receive long-term opioid prescriptions than Black patients, leading to more prescription opioid addiction.[2]

The other variable that makes it difficult to make sense of the opioid crisis's demographics is the fact that they have changed significantly over time, and since the opioid crisis is ongoing, they could continue to change in the future. While initially the opioid crisis largely involved the abuse of prescription opioids, over time the increased regulation of prescription opioids combined with the increased availability and low price of illegal opioids like heroin and fentanyl have changed the demographic landscape. The opioid crisis was originally thought to be a health issue that primarily impacted poor and working-class white Americans living in rural areas. Working-class people in rural areas tended to be prescribed opioids at higher rates and often had to travel a great distance for opioid addiction treatment, which contributed to higher rates of addiction in these populations.[3] However, once there was a rise in the use of heroin and other illegal opioids, urban populations—especially Black people and other people of color—started to see a dramatic rise in addiction and overdose rates.[4] Receiving adequate health care for opioid addiction was also a struggle in marginalized urban communities, though for different reasons.

The viewpoints in this chapter take a look at research findings about which groups of Americans have felt the greatest impacts of this crisis. They examine the economic and sociological reasons for these differences. In grappling with these questions they are also forced to reckon with their complexity and constantly evolving nature.

Notes

1. Carla R. Jackson, "Addressing the Opioid Crisis in Urban America," Morgan State University, 2020. https://magazine.morgan.edu/addressing-the-opioid-crisis-in-urban-america/.
2. Claudia López Lloreda, "In the Same Health System, Black Patients Are Prescribed Fewer Opioids than White Patients," *STAT News*, July 21, 2021. https://www.

statnews.com/2021/07/21/black-patients-prescribed-fewer-opioids-white-patients/.

3. Clark Merrefield, "'Deaths of Despair': Research on Opioid Crisis Origins and the Link Between Minimum Wages and Suicide Reduction," *Journalist's Resource*, January 19, 2022. https://journalistsresource.org/economics/deaths-of-despair-opioid-minimum-wage-suicide/.

4. Richard Florida, "The Changing Geography of the Opioid Crisis," *Bloomberg CityLab*, December 5, 2019. https://www.bloomberg.com/news/articles/2019-12-05/how-opioid-deaths-differ-in-rural-and-urban-areas.

> *"Compared with their urban counterparts, rural communities face significant barriers to treatment, such as fewer facilities, which may also offer more limited services, and greater distances to care."*

Rural Communities Are Hit Particularly Hard by the Opioid Crisis

Pew Charitable Trusts

People in rural areas who develop an addiction to opioids face a distinct set of challenges compared to their urban counterparts, which have caused the overdose death rates in rural communities to skyrocket during the opioid crisis. According to this viewpoint, opioid prescription rates have historically been higher in rural parts of the U.S., and it has been more difficult for people in these areas to access effective opioid treatment. Often, patients in these areas will be offered fewer treatment options than patients who live in cities, and they may have to travel a great distance to access the treatments that are available. The Pew Charitable Trusts is a nonprofit, non-governmental organization that conducts research to inform public policy.

As you read, consider the following questions:

1. How much did overdose deaths increase in rural areas between 1999 and 2015?

2. What are some of the barriers to treatment for opioid addiction that are listed in the viewpoint?

3. At the time this viewpoint was published, what percentage of large rural counties lacked opioid treatment programs (OTPs)?

The increasing number of drug overdose deaths in the United States has hit rural areas particularly hard. Between 1999 and 2015, overdose deaths increased 325 percent in rural counties.[1] In 2015, they surpassed the death rate in urban areas.[2] Additionally, nonfatal prescription opioid overdoses are concentrated in states with large rural populations.[3] Helping to drive this trend in rural areas are high opioid prescription rates and challenges accessing medication-assisted treatment (MAT), the gold standard for treating opioid use disorder.[4]

This fact sheet describes some of the challenges rural communities face in providing access to evidence-based treatment and strategies used by federal and state agencies to enhance treatment capacity, including how one rural community responded to the opioid epidemic by addressing the specific needs of its residents. The policies and programs described are not an exhaustive list but are intended to be illustrative.

Medication-assisted treatment (MAT) combines behavioral therapy with one of three Food and Drug Administration (FDA)-approved medications—buprenorphine, methadone, or naltrexone—for the treatment of opioid use disorder (OUD).[5]

These medications minimize or block the euphoric effects of opioids, curtail cravings, and significantly increase a patient's adherence to treatment.[6]

Rural Treatment Capacity

Compared with their urban counterparts, rural communities face significant barriers to treatment, such as fewer facilities, which may also offer more limited services, and greater distances to care.[7]

Opioid treatment programs (OTPs), which dispense methadone and may also offer buprenorphine and naltrexone, are a key component of most current opioid use disorder (OUD) treatment systems. Although a shortage of these programs exists nationally, the gap is widest in rural areas, where 88.6 percent of large rural counties lack a sufficient number of OTPs.[8]

> An opioid treatment program (OTP) is a facility where patients go, usually daily, to take medications to treat their OUD under the supervision of staff and to receive counseling and other care services.
>
> These programs are regulated and certified by the federal Substance Abuse and Mental Health Services Administration and operate in a number of care settings, including intensive outpatient, residential, and hospital locations.[9]

Another key component of an OUD treatment system is office-based opioid treatment (OBOT), which integrates opioid agonist treatment (i.e., drugs that minimize the effects of opioids) into a patient's general medical and psychiatric regimen by allowing primary care physicians to provide MAT in their own clinical settings.[10] However, OBOT is particularly limited in rural communities: 29.8 percent of rural Americans live in a county without a buprenorphine provider, compared with only 2.2 percent of urban Americans.[11]

The shortage of treatment options in rural areas places barriers on patients who must travel farther to access MAT and, in some cases, have to rely on friends or family for transportation.[12] Numerous studies have found that those who live closer to a health care facility have better health outcomes and can more easily access care.[13] Transportation challenges may be particularly acute for patients with OUD; a small survey of OTP patients in Vermont found that 23 percent missed at least one visit due to lack of transportation, 17 percent due to weather, and 8 percent due to costs.[14] The rural treatment shortage also places burdens on payers that offer patients transportation services.[15] For example, Washington state's Medicaid program reported in 2011 that it spends $3 million a year to transport rural enrollees of the program to urban OTPs.[16]

Treatment centers in rural areas are less likely than their urban counterparts to provide buprenorphine and to offer additional services, such as case management, that are shown to improve outcomes.[17] Rural facilities also rely more on public funds to care for patients and support innovative programs that may improve treatment quality.[18] Such limitations can contribute to decreased availability of evidence-based care, with fewer tailored treatment options and specialized providers to address complex patients.

Closing the Treatment Gap by Expanding the Provider Workforce

In 2016, Congress passed legislation temporarily allowing nurse practitioners (NPs) and physician assistants (PAs) to prescribe buprenorphine after completing specified training.[19] Additional legislation passed in 2018 made this allowance permanent and temporarily authorized other providers, such as clinical nurse specialists, to obtain a waiver to become buprenorphine prescribers.[20] This expanded prescribing authority is relevant for rural areas; in 2017, 13.8 percent of rural counties had a waivered NP and 4.6 percent had a waivered PA.[21] As a result of this workforce expansion—and a 10.7 percent rise in the number of physicians with a waiver to prescribe buprenorphine—from 2012 to 2017, the number of all waivered providers (e.g., physicians, NPs, and PAs) per 100,000 residents doubled in rural counties.

However, as of 2017, 28 states prohibited NPs from prescribing buprenorphine unless they are working in collaboration with a doctor who also has a federal waiver to prescribe.[22] To further increase access to MAT, states may need to change laws and regulations that restrict NPs from prescribing buprenorphine.

Using Technology to Address Physician Barriers

For rural physicians, barriers to prescribing buprenorphine include time constraints and a lack of mental health or psychosocial support services for patients, specialty backup for complex problems, and confidence in their ability to manage OUD.[23] Treatment models that use technology to address these barriers have been shown to increase access in rural populations.

For example, Project ECHO (Extension for Community Healthcare Outcomes), which was launched in New Mexico, contributed to a nearly tenfold increase in buprenorphine-waivered physicians over a 10-year period.[24] In this model, prescribers are recruited to obtain a waiver and are provided regular opportunities for mentoring and education, thereby increasing treatment capacity in rural areas.

West Virginia's Comprehensive Opioid Addiction Treatment program is a telemedicine model that uses videoconferencing to prescribe buprenorphine and for medication management.[25] Patients residing hundreds of miles from the treatment center participate in virtual group-based medication management followed by in-person group therapy. Retrospective analysis of this program found that rates of treatment retention and abstinence from drug use were comparable to the rates observed when MAT is provided in person.

Developing Innovative, Local Responses to the Opioid Epidemic

Strategies to address the opioid epidemic must address community needs to effectively reach and treat patients with OUD. For example, Indiana's Scott County Partnership Inc. responded to an HIV outbreak that was linked to the misuse of prescription opioids and sharing of syringes by developing a "one-stop shop" model to provide buprenorphine, mental health counseling, HIV and hepatitis C treatment, primary care, and syringe exchange in an existing mental health clinic.[26] Prior to this model, this rural county had no OUD or HIV treatment services.[27]

Scott County responded to this local public health crisis by comprehensively addressing the barriers to care faced by people with OUD and HIV. In addition to health care services, patients receive clothes and meals if needed, obtain help finding a job, and have care coordinators to help them enroll in health insurance.[28] The partnership also transports patients to appointments and conducts outreach and education to increase the number of physicians who can prescribe buprenorphine.[29] Evaluations of the one-stop shop model have not been published, although Scott County's experience provides an example of a targeted response that takes specific community needs into account.

Closing the Rural Treatment Gap

Policymakers and leaders within health care systems can ensure that effective OUD therapy is available in rural communities by implementing emerging and evidence-based practices and studying the effectiveness of these models within their states. These efforts can help close the treatment gap in rural America and save lives.

Endnotes

1. Karin A. Mack, Christopher M. Jones, and Michael F. Ballesteros, "Illicit Drug Use, Illicit Drug Use Disorders, and Drug Overdose Deaths in Metropolitan and Nonmetropolitan Areas—United States," Morbidity and Mortality Weekly Report 66, no. 19 (2017): 1-12, https://www.cdc.gov/mmwr/volumes/66/ss/ss6619a1.htm?s_cid=ss6619a1_w. The 325 percent increase in overdose deaths is an age-adjusted calculation, meaning it allows for the comparison of communities with different age structures.

2. Ibid.

3. Katherine M. Keyes et al., "Understanding the Rural-Urban Differences in Nonmedical Prescription Opioid Use and Abuse in the United States," American Journal of Public Health 104, no. 2 (2014): e52-59, https://www.ncbi.nlm.nih.gov/pmc/articles/PMC3935688.

4. Ibid.; Roger Rosenblatt et al., "Geographic and Specialty Distribution of US Physicians Trained to Treat Opioid Use Disorder," Annals of Family Medicine 13, no. 1 (2015): 23-6, https://dx.doi.org/10.1370%2Fafm.1735; Substance Abuse and Mental Health Services Administration, "Addressing Substance Use and the Opioid Epidemic in Integrated Care Settings" (PowerPoint, Primary and Behavioral Health Care Integration Central Regional Meeting, Denver, March 8-9, 2018), https://integration.samhsa.gov/pbhci-learning-community/regional_clusters/Hamblin.Disselkoen.Mountain_Plains.ATTC_PBHCI_SUD_Presentation.pdf.

5. American Society of Addiction Medicine, "The ASAM National Practice Guideline for the Use of Medications in the Treatment of Addiction Involving Opioid Use" (2015), http://www.asam.org/docs/default-source/practice-support/guidelines-and-consensus-docs/asam-national-practice-guideline-supplement.pdf?sfvrsn=24; U.S. Department of Health and Human Services, "Addressing Prescription Drug Abuse in the United States: Current Activities and Future Opportunities" (2013), https://www.cdc.gov/drugoverdose/pdf/hhs_prescription_drug_abuse_report_09.2013.pdf.

6. Richard P. Mattick et al., "Methadone Maintenance Therapy Versus No Opioid Replacement Therapy for Opioid Dependence," Cochrane Database of Systematic Reviews no. 3 (2009), https://doi.org/10.1002/14651858.CD002209.pub2.

7. Ellen Pullen and Carrie Oser, "Barriers to Substance Abuse Treatment in Rural and Urban Communities: A Counselor Perspective," Substance Use & Misuse 49, no. 7 (2014): 891-901, http://dx.doi.org/10.3109/10826084.2014.891615; Quentin Johnson, Brian Mund, and Paul J. Joudrey, "Improving Rural Access to Opioid Treatment Programs," Journal of Law, Medicine & Ethics 46, no. 2 (2018): 437-39, https://doi.org/10.1177/1073110518782951.

8. Andrew W. Dick et al., "Growth in Buprenorphine Waivers for Physicians Increased Potential Access to Opioid Agonist Treatment, 200211," Health Affairs 34, no. 6 (2015): 1028-34, https://dx.doi.org/10.1377%2Fhlthaff.2014.1205.

9. U.S. Department of Health and Human Services, "Medication-Assisted Treatment for Opioid Addiction in Opioid Treatment Programs: Inservice Training" (2008, reprinted 2009), http://www.woema.org/pdf/WOHC2013PDF/SAMHSA-Med-Assist%20tx%20for%20opioid%20addiction.pdf.

10. American Society of Addiction Medicine, "Public Policy Statement on Office-Based Opioid Agonist Treatment (OBOT)," (2010), https://www.asam.org/docs/default-source/public-policy-statements/1obot-treatment-7-04.pdf?sfvrsn=0.

11. C. Holly A. Andrilla et al., "Geographic Distribution of Providers With a DEA Waiver to Prescribe Buprenorphine for the Treatment of Opioid Use Disorder: A 5-Year Update," The Journal of Rural Health 35, no. 1 (2018): 108-12, https://doi.org/10.1111/jrh.12307.

12. Andrew Rosenblum et al., "Distance Traveled and Cross-State Commuting to Opioid Treatment Programs in the United States," Journal of Environmental and Public Health (2011): 1-10, http://dx.doi.org/10.1155/2011/948789; Stacey C. Sigmon, "Access to Treatment for Opioid Dependence in Rural America: Challenges and Future Directions," JAMA Psychiatry 71, no. 4 (2014): 359-60, http://dx.doi.org/10.1001/jamapsychiatry.2013.4450; Pullen and Oser, "Barriers to Substance Abuse Treatment."

13. Charlotte Kelly et al., "Are Differences in Travel Time or Distance to Healthcare for Adults in Global North Countries Associated With an Impact on Health Outcomes? A Systematic Review," BMJ Open 6, no. 11 (2016): 1-9, http://dx.doi.org/10.1136/bmjopen-2016-013059.

14. Sigmon, "Access to Treatment."

15. Erik Kvamme et al., "Who Prescribes Buprenorphine for Rural Patients? The Impact of Specialty, Location and Practice Type in Washington State," Journal of Substance Abuse Treatment 44, no. 3 (2013): 355-60, https://dx.doi.org/10.1016%2Fj.jsat.2012.07.006.

16. Ibid

17. Mary Bond Edmond, Lydia Aletraris, and Paul M. Roman, "Rural Substance Use Treatment Centers in the United States: An Assessment of Treatment Quality by

Location," American Journal of Drug and Alcohol Abuse 41, no. 5 (2015): 449-57, https://dx.doi.org/10.3109%2F00952990.2015.1059842.

18. Ibid.

19. Comprehensive Addiction and Recovery Act, sec. 303: Medication-Assisted Treatment for Recovery From Addiction (2016), https://www.congress.gov/bill/114th-congress/senate-bill/524/text.

20. Substance Use Disorder Prevention That Promotes Opioid Recovery and Treatment for Patients and Communities Act, sec. 3201: Allowing for More Flexibility With Respect to Medication-Assisted Treatment for Opioid Use Disorders (2018), https://www.congress.gov/115/bills/hr6/BILLS-115hr6enr.pdf.

21. Andrilla et al., "Geographic Distribution of Providers."

22. Christine Vestal, "Nurse Licensing Laws Block Treatment for Opioid Addiction," Stateline (April 21, 2017), accessed Aug. 28, 2018, http://www.pewtrusts.org/en/research-and-analysis/blogs/stateline/2017/04/21/nurse-licensing-laws-block-treatment-for-opioid-addiction.

23. C. Holly A. Andrilla, Cynthia Coulthard, and Eric H. Larson, "Barriers Rural Physicians Face Prescribing Buprenorphine for Opioid Use Disorder," Annals of Family Medicine 15, no. 4 (2017): 359-62, http://dx.doi.org/10.1370/afm.2099.

24. Miriam Komaromy et al., "Project ECHO (Extension for Community Healthcare Outcomes): A New Model for Educating Primary Care Providers About Treatment of Substance Use Disorders," Substance Abuse 37, no. 1 (2016): 20-4, http://dx.doi.org/10.1080/08897077.2015.1129388.

25. Wanhong Zheng et al., "Treatment Outcome Comparison Between Telepsychiatry and Face-to-Face Buprenorphine Medication-Assisted Treatment for Opioid Use Disorder: A 2-Year Retrospective Data Analysis," Journal of Addiction Medicine 11, no. 2 (2017): 138-44, http://dx.doi.org/10.1097/ADM.0000000000000287.

26. Ibid.; P. Todd Korthuis et al., "Primary Care-Based Models for the Treatment of Opioid Use Disorder: A Scoping Review," Annals of Internal Medicine 166, no. 4 (2017): 268-78, https://dx.doi.org/10.7326%2FM16-2149.

27. Ibid.

28. Michelle Goodin, Scott County Health Department, pers. comm. to The Pew Charitable Trusts, Nov. 20, 2018.

29. Elizabeth Beilman, "State-Ordered 'One-Stop Shop' for HIV Outbreak Open in Scott County," News and Tribune, April 1, 2015, https://www.newsandtribune.com/news/state-ordered-one-stop-shop-for-hiv-outbreak-open-in/article_31572476-d8d7-11e4-9aad-33610ed3dbd0.html; Korthuis et al., "Primary Care-Based Models"; Goodin, pers. comm.

> *"As with most societal ills in this country, the current epidemic of opioid addiction has made a deeper impact on the marginalized, the poor and those whom mainstream society judges most harshly."*

The Effect of the Opioid Crisis on Urban Populations Has Been Ignored

Carla R. Jackson

In the following viewpoint Carla R. Jackson argues that although the opioid crisis is often considered an issue that mainly effects white people in rural and suburban areas, urban Black communities are being devastated by opioids as well, and their struggles are going largely ignored. Marginalized urban communities facing homelessness, poverty, and addiction in cities have a hard time accessing treatment for opioid addiction and often face harsher judgment for their addiction. Morgan State University's School of Social Work is trying to prepare social workers who are entering the field to address the urban opioid crisis. Carla R. Jackson is a freelance higher education consultant based in Baltimore, Maryland.

"Addressing the Opioid Crisis in Urban America," by Carla R. Jackson, Morgan State University. Reprinted by permission.

As you read, consider the following questions:

1. According to Carla R. Jackson, what are the challenges faced by professionals who treat opioid addiction in urban communities?
2. What has Morgan State University's School of Social Work done to help prepare students to address urban opioid addiction?
3. What are some of the other issues that addiction intersects with, according to Laurens Van Sluytman?

The tremendous increase in addiction and deaths caused by opiates over the past few years has changed the name and public face of the problem in the United States. The suffering of white, suburban Americans now figures prominently in the narrative of what is now known as "the opioid crisis," however, the African-American, urban community has also experienced a significant increase in opioid deaths. Moreover, as with most societal ills in this country, the current epidemic of opioid addiction has made a deeper impact on the marginalized, the poor and those whom mainstream society judges most harshly.

"Addiction intersects with homelessness, poverty, mental illness and high-risk behaviors outside of substance abuse. There is survival sex and other types of behaviors that are in the service of the addiction," said Laurens Van Sluytman, Ph.D., LCSW, assistant dean and associate professor in Morgan State University's (MSU's) School of Social Work.

The lack of access to treatment and rehabilitation for those affected in urban, African-American communities, and the lack of research and limited funding to address the problem there, have long challenged professionals serving the needs of these communities. These practitioners often fill the gap left by policies and public health campaigns that do not fully consider the areas' cultural and historical nuances.

Since its founding, Morgan's School of Social Work has been fully vested in its institutional mission to serve urban communities through a wide variety of social, economic and social justice initiatives. And under the direction of its dean, Anna McPhatter, Ph.D., the school has a long history of work with addiction. Of the more than 500 social work degree programs across the nation, the MSU undergraduate program is one of only four that require students to take a course in chemical dependence. That requirement has been a part of the curriculum for more than 25 years. Faculty have built on that foundation in recent years by creating a concentration in addiction, including required courses in treatment, pharmacology and social work ethics focused on working with people with addictions or addictive behaviors.

"Our students have to be well-trained and deeply immersed in our ethics as social workers to approach these problems and these populations in a nonjudgmental space, in order to provide the services and the linkages, and the engagement and assessment," said Dr. Van Sluytman. "It is difficult for people to sit sometimes with someone who has an open abscess, right?"

Moving the Needle

On any given day, at least 250 MSU social work students are serving as interns in agencies in Baltimore City, providing approximately 300,000 hours of free service annually, valued at about $7 million. Dr. Van Sluytman noted that although the goal of the internships is to educate students, their work must also inform the field.

"We have to be sure that our students are driven by data," he explained. "What works? How long does it take to work?

What are the most effective interventions for this community?"

Many Morgan social work graduates return to the communities from which they hail, trained to advocate for and understand the cultural dynamics of the neighborhoods they serve.

"The epidemic (of opioid addiction) in our community is very different from what is being televised. Our students know our

U.S. Drug Overdose Deaths Surpass 100,000 in 2021

Drug overdose deaths in the United States exceeded 100,000 in the 12-month period ending last April, a record number, according to provisional data from the CDC. The data shows that there were an estimated 100,306 overdose deaths nationwide during those 12 months, up from 78,056 reported during the same period last year, an increase of 28.5%.

Synthetic opioids, especially fentanyl, continued to be the leading reason for overdose deaths, accounting for nearly two-thirds (64%) of all overdose deaths, an increase of 49% from the previous year.

The CDC notes that fentanyl is 50 times stronger than morphine and heroin, and is often sold illegally because it has similar effects to heroin.

These figures show that overdose deaths from methamphetamine and other psychostimulants also grew significantly, up 48% in the year ending April 2021 compared to the previous year.

Deaths from cocaine and prescription painkillers were also up from the previous year, but not as dramatically.

After learning that data, President Joe Biden pledged to do everything in his "power to address addiction and end the overdose epidemic."

"We are strengthening prevention, promoting harm reduction, expanding treatment, and supporting people in recovery, as well as reducing the supply of harmful substances in our communities. And we won't let up," Biden said.

**"Drug Crisis: Overdose Deaths Surpass 100,000 for First Time in U.S. History,"
El American, November 18, 2021.**

community, and they know the history of our community," said Dr. Van Sluytman. "That is what urban social work is about."

Dr. McPhatter echoed Dr. Van Sluytman's thought that cultural awareness and sensitivity are pivotal in urban environments: "In general, the focus we've given to drugs, drug use and drug violence in our curriculum absolutely makes our students…more efficient at calming a situation down to get the information they need to assess and refer, without calling the police."

Co-principal Investigators Anthony Estreet, Ph.D., and Taqi Tirmazi, Ph.D., associate professors in the School of Social Work, recently received a $1.3-million grant from the Health Resources and Services Administration (HRSA) to develop an initiative titled Graduate Interns Future Trends (G.I.F.T.). G.I.F.T. provides specialized training in mental health and substance abuse to 90 Master of Social Work (M.S.W.) students to prepare them to address the addiction epidemic facing the city of Baltimore and other urban areas. Students received $10,000 stipends to complete the training, and the School of Social Work developed extensive collaborations with community-based agencies to enhance their training. In addition, Dr. Estreet's expertise in substance use disorders has evolved into a partnership with the federal Substance Abuse and Mental Health Administration (SAMHSA) and its Region 3 Addiction Technology Transfer Center, to provide ongoing training to community agencies and students.

To meet the goals of these initiatives, Dr. Estreet is conducting research that addresses treatment outcomes in the minority population.

"We have created the Health and Addiction Research Training Lab, which allows us to partner with M.S.W. and Ph.D. students to conduct research and to document the efforts that we are engaging in around the issues that are specifically related to addiction."

Reflecting on the work that still needs to be done in this field, Dr. McPhatter raised Morgan's obligation and responsibility to Baltimore.

"We've got to be the people at the table," she said. "We have to develop the models, the plans and the interventions to move the needle on these challenges. As an urban research institution and an anchor university in this city, we must play a significant role in altering the narrative and trajectory of the critical issues facing our city."

"Drug overdose by race increased among Blacks in the urban settings by 41% in 2016, which outpaced any other race or ethnic group."

Opioid Addiction Has a Devastating Effect on Black Communities

Clairmont Griffith, Bernice La France, Clayton Bacchus, and Gezzer Ortega

In the following viewpoint, Clairmont Griffith, Bernice La France, Clayton Bacchus, and Gezzer Ortega argue that opioid addiction has affected the Black American population disproportionately. Lack of equal resources has led to higher rates of incarceration and death, affecting Black American families to a degree that will likely impact several generations to follow. Clairmont Griffith and Bernice La France are affiliated with the Department of Anesthesiology at Howard University College of Medicine. Clayton Bacchus is with Inner City Family Services in Affiliation with Howard University Hospital. Gezzer Ortega, MD, MPH is affiliated with Brigham and Women's Hospital and an instructor at Harvard Medical School.

As you read, consider the following questions:

1. According to data cited in this viewpoint, in which states were rates of fatal overdose by Blacks nearly double those of whites?
2. How does lack of representation hurt the Black community when it comes to opioids?
3. What has drug overdose replaced as the leading cause of death in America, according to the authors?

The United States grapples with one of its worst drug crises; the country loses more than 800 people each week from opioid-related overdoses. Drug overdose by race increased among Blacks in the urban settings by 41% in 2016, which outpaced any other race or ethnic group [1]. Drug overdose is a critical health issue in the country exceeding heart diseases in causing deaths among different races of the American population [2]. Opioid disorders have resulted in the recent advances such as rehabilitation programs, public health interventions, and treatment programs. Policymakers have designed various approaches to the opioid crisis in efforts to increase war on drugs and crackdowns on crime. The anti-drug trafficking programs emerged to address the new opioid addiction rates, which are growing among the Black Communities [3]. Widespread drug use has dumped the country into deaths attributed to pharmaceutical opioids such as heroin that accounted for 19 per cent of overdose deaths in 2013 [3]. According to the New England Journal of Medicine, opioid addiction leads to public health risks [3]. Volkow and McLellan's research reflects on the scope of the epidemic among the Caucasian which exceeded Blacks' because minority races received under treatment for years. A similar study by JAMA in 2008 found that minority races are not likely to receive opioids for pain in an emergency department compared to the majority [2]. As a result, it is possible that pills would be sold on the streets to Black patients. Despite stepped efforts to address the crisis, health experts say that overdose deaths keep climbing each year, especially among the Black race. Moreover, the office of Medical Examiner in Washington D.C reported that opioid overdose deaths among men aged 40 to 69 moved up in the period between 2014 and 2017 [4]. Whereas previous data show that the drug addiction crisis started in rural America among the Caucasians, the overall opioid overdose death has increased among the Black community leading to a high number of deaths [4].

Methodology

This chapter provides details of the secondary methods used in effects of opioids research on the Black Community. The study obtained information from various sources such as libraries, local bodies, and Literature review and government websites. The Secondary research was vital for this study since existing information was highly useful in determining results.

Methods

The study utilised a secondary analysis of existing data, with research "question driven" and "data-driven" approaches [5]. The two methods are significant in this paper as they focused on already existing data. The existing data used scholarly resources consisting of private and public information. There is an array of existing public data that address specific topics on effects of opioid addiction on health-related databases. Specifically, the research targeted existing data, and county and regional levels in the United States. The government websites provide up to date information related to opioid addiction in the US with the latest being 2016 statistics [4]. Variety of US-based government agencies offer online data with well-analysed frequencies and cross-tabulations. As a result, websites offer technical support that aided identification of potential data sources in the systems. The specific data provided current statistics on mortality and an array of health conditions related to opioid addiction.

While employing both questions-driven and data-driven methods for analysing existing data, the research considered possible variables for the research question. It implies that a comprehensive understanding of the credibility of data sources was employed to design quality control measures to assess information [5]. The chosen documents contained sufficient information with meaningful estimates about opioid addiction among members of the Black community. Before conducting the analysis, it was possible to generate outcome and confounding variables which were used during the review. The methods helped the research to recode original variables to meet the assumptions in the research question. Moreover, the secondary data research focused on the opioid addiction conditions.

Discussion

Death Rates of Opioids According to Race

The number of Blacks dying from opioid has reached an extended rate higher than the general population in numerous states such as Missouri, Illinois, Minnesota, Wisconsin, West Virginia and Washington, D.C. [6]. For instance, death rates in the states of Virginia and Wisconsin have numbers of Blacks with fatal overdose rate nearly double that of Caucasians. On the other hand, Illinois is the best example of effects of opioid epidemic among the Blacks. According to data from the Illinois Department of Public Health, all opioid deaths in the state doubled among Blacks than any other racial group during the period from 2013 to 2016 with a 132% increase.4 Despite making up to 15% of the Illinois population, Blacks account for about one-quarter of opioid overdose deaths. While the country focuses on rural areas for opioid addicts, the trend has shifted to urban areas which currently experience the crisis from day-to-day [7]. Chicago alone has had an extreme increase in a fatal opioid overdose, which sharply increased to 75%. In Chicago, Blacks make approximately 32% of the population, but they account for about half of all opioid deaths which are 48.4%. In 2016, the rate of African American deaths was 56% which was higher than Caucasians' death rate from opioids. Consequently,

CDC data reveals that the 2016 Black's death in Chicago was almost four times higher than the national average rate in 2015.

The Most Affected States with Opioid Addiction

Majority of the Blacks with opioid addiction come from the low-income families and rarely receive treatment, unlike the Caucasians who share these characteristics but end up enrolled to private insurances [7]. With little access to evidence-based treatment, the Black community has more people dying from opioid addiction epidemic. In fact, data show that the majority of Blacks live in Chicago however; the state has the lowest treatment capacity for buprenorphine. That is, Chicago is the third most depressed cities in the national rank such capacity rate makes services less available for Blacks in need of treatment.

The data presented in Table 1 shows that the states with more opioid-related cases have the highest numbers of Blacks living in the respective cities. It is a clear that Blacks are dying at a higher rate impacted by the epidemic which is a higher proportion than the general US population [7]. The top ten most affected States with the opioid crisis are in Midwest; they include Missouri, Wisconsin, Illinois, and Minnesota among others (Table 2). For example, Illinois alone has an opioid death rate for Blacks of 11.6 per 100,000 in 2015, compared to 10.4 for the general population. In some cases, some states had Blacks' opioid overdose rate exceeding other races. For example, Missouri and Wisconsin have 14.8 per 100,000 and 21.9 per 100,000 respectively [6]. Besides, other areas such as West Virginia have Black's overdose rates that doubled that of the Caucasian. Most Blacks face significant barriers that hinder them from accessing care; these issues include living in racially concentrated areas, lack of insurance, childcare, transportation issues and other issues. However, these issue not only do they affect the Blacks' living in poverty but also the Caucasians. The main contributors to lower life expectancies are the health disparities among Blacks [4].

Table 1: Major United States cities and corresponding counties by Buprenorphine treatment capacity, 2015.

RANK	CITY	COUNTY	COUNTY POPULATION	TREATMENT CAPACITY (N)	CAPACITY (RATE/100,000)
1	PHILADELPHIA, PA	PHILADELPHIA	1,526,006	12,570	824
2	NEW YORK, NY	MULTIPLE	8,175,133	63,840	781
3	SAN DIEGO, CA	SAN DIEGO	3,095,313	15,970	516
4	PHOENIX, AZ	MARICOPA	3,817,117	15,040	394
5	SAN JOSE, CA	SANTA CLARA	1,781,642	6,630	372
6	LOS ANGELES, CA	LOS ANGELES	9,818,605	33,510	341
7	HOUSTON, TX	HARRIS	4,092,459	12,780	312
8	CHICAGO, IL	COOK	5,194,675	15,360	296
9	DALLAS, TX	DALLAS	2,368,139	6,820	288
10	SAN ANTONIO, TX	BEXAR	1,714,773	4,810	281

Data source: Illinois Department of Public Health, Cook County Medical Examiner's Office, US Census Bureau.

Table 2: Top 10 States with the highest rate of opioid overdose deaths 2015.

STATE	WHITE	AFRICAN AMERICAN	GENERAL POPULATION
WESTERN VIRGINIA	36.2	55.5	36
DISTRICT OF COLUMBIA	NR	22.8	14.5
WISCONSIN	11.3	21.9	11.2
OHIO	27.7	15.2	24.7
MARYLAND	25	14.8	17.7
MISSOURI	11.9	14.8	17.7
MASSACHUSETTS	27.1	13.2	23.3
MICHIGAN	14.7	12.4	13.6
ILLINOIS	13.1	11.6	10.7
MINNESOTA	6	10	6.2
UNITED STATES	13.9	6.6	10.4

Data Source: Cook County Medical Examiner's Office, US Census Bureau.

Comparison Between Chicago and Illinois in Opioid Addiction

Illinois: Table 3 presents excellent examples of how overdose rates related to opioids hit Black populations [6]. For instance, these cases increased in Illinois by 82% which corresponds to data from the Illinois Department for Public health that shows opioid deaths (heroin and pain pills) escalated faster among the Blacks more than any other race from 2013 to 2016 [6]. Similarly, the period saw Black deaths from pain pills increasing to about three times the increase in the Caucasian fatalities. In other words, the Black community around the country have been stricken by the effects of opioid addiction, and continue to suffer.

Table 3: Illinois fatal overdoses from any opioid from 2013-2016.

RACIAL GROUP	2013	2014	2015	2016	% CHANGE
WHITE	758	876	1,029	1,230	62%
AFRICAN AMERICAN	198	229	235	459	132%
OTHER	12	7	8	24	100%
LATINO	104	91	110	204	96%
TOTAL	1,072	1,203	1,382	1,946	82%

Data source: Cook County Medical Examiner's Office, US Census Bureau.

Chicago: Chicago has had higher overdose rates in Black communities involving heroin, Fentanyl, and other opioids [8]. The effects of addiction are prevalent in the South and West sides, but Austin suffers the highest death rate than all the community areas. Chicago suffers from the high addiction of fentanyl-adulterated heroin, whose deaths represent 58% of opioid deaths in 2016, thrice deaths accounted for in 2015 [8]. Some of the highest overdose regions include North Lawndale, East, and West Garfield Park, Austin, Fuller Park, Humboldt and Englewood. All listed areas are made up of poverty concentrated areas, which are located in the South and West zones of Chicago [8].

Challenges of Opioid Addiction on the Black Community

The opioid epidemic has a social effect that leaves communities with visible impacts. Firstly, the problem has led to family disintegration especially with the massive rise in cracking down for drug addiction. It has emerged that the US government and judicial systems display matters of racial stereotypes as they try to fight drug use crisis [9]. Numerous data show the opiate issues have irreparably harmed the Black American youth. The opiate crisis has continuously pushed the Black community into devastation and crisis of incarceration, separating them from the rest of family members [7]. Notably, war on drugs policies is misused by the law enforcement authorities that target Black neighborhood. Initially, war on drugs declaration aimed at taking a stand on corrupt government members and criminal organizations that can deter the country from lucrative drug market [2]. In reality, these wars target Black communities, whereby law enforcement disproportionately focuses on people of color for drug violations. Previous studies show that despite drug use being similar between Caucasian and Blacks, Blacks have 13 times more chances to be arrested for buying, and using drugs.4 However, in some states, rates are higher. For instance, Black and Hispanic population in 2013 represented 29 per cent of the US population however; they dominated in numbers of prisoners for drug offenses [10]. The US Sentencing Commission revealed that Blacks received longer prison sentences for drug-related offenses than other races in the country despite being convicted for crimes of similar weight. Bureau of Justice Statistics proves that in 2012, state prisons had 225,242 inmates for drug-related offenses [10]. However, 45% of inmates were Black and 30% Caucasian. Such statistics is an attribution of how often police were likely to arrest addicts in low-income ethnic minority neighborhoods. As stated earlier, Cooks County Illinois has 5.24 million residents, while a quarter of the population are Blacks. However, Black population represent more than 70% of the county's incarcerated population [10]. Consequently, those arrested are from low-income families, with low levels of education and have negligible job prospects. Most of these victims have a mental problem and might have had a history of childhood abuse and trauma. Besides, opioid addicts rarely have a stable family or social network on which they can rely but have offspring to support.

Another consequence of Black American addiction is lack of adequate representation to argue for reduced charges compared to other races [9]. As a result, Black Americans quickly get arrested and convicted due to the little resources to secure competent legal defense. Previous studies have proved that the United States is a race-based institution where only the Black Americans are arrested more often than Caucasian Americans for the same characteristics of drug-related offenses [6]. In 2000, New York City had arrested more addicts among Black Americans than Caucasians in four other states. Usually, police stopped and frisked young Black males, and when arrested, Blacks have to endure long waits in prisons before they receive a trial. Detailed investigation of the criminal justice system indicated that a high profile killing of the Black youth was made by police officers from other ethnic backgrounds [11]. For instance, the 2014 and 2015 report revealed that most lawyers and police officers in the US are of Caucasian origin. According to American Bar Associations reports, 88% of its lawyers are white while 4.8% are Blacks [11]. It indicates that Black Americans are exposed to more risks than Caucasian, which leads them to 10 times chances of arrest higher than those among the Caucasian.

Government Actions to Help Opioid Addicted People

In a report prepared by Roster of commissioners, the Federal government has programs directed towards prevention and treatment of the drug-related activities [11]. The Federal government has a recommendable history in developing evidence-based programs and policies that aim at reducing the number of people affected by opioids nationwide. Besides, the national government has launched prevention campaigns to address the use and abuse of illicit drugs as an alternative to prevent premature and preventable deaths or disabilities. There are national campaigns focused on opioids' risks and consequences, educating families on the warning signs, and channelling the message to specific populations such as elderly, college students, adolescent and pregnant women. Furthermore, the government has also reviewed the medical school's curricula to ensure that practitioners are trained to conduct proper prescription as a vital strategy to address the opioid epidemic [11]. Therefore, the government has set aside budgetary allocations to support Drug-Impaired Driving program, Anti-doping activities and Prevention research among others [12].

Limitations

Generally, secondary analysis of the existing data in its nature fails to address the particular research question. As viewed in the discussion, the data was not collected for the entire population subgroups for all regions in the United States. There is a probability that most crucial information on the zip codes and names if the primary sampling responded were omitted. Another major limitation of analysing the existing data is that the researcher is not the same person who conducted the primary data collection process. Therefore, it is probably right that the data may have specific glitches in the data collection process which may hinder the interpretation of the particular variables in the data. It is therefore hard to provide succinct documentation of valuable information presented in the document because the user may not show relevance in the submitted data.

Conclusion

Drug overdose by race is a recent issue among the Black Community. These rates have escalated sharply among the Blacks in urban settings. For instance, some related opioid effects rose among the Blacks by 41% in 2016 outpacing any other race or ethnic group. As a result, drug overdose has become a significant health issue in the country surpassing heart illnesses as the leading cause of deaths among the different races of the American population. Opioid disorders have resulted in the recent advances in rehabilitation programs, public health interventions, and treatments programs. Numerous data show that opiate issues have irreparably harmed the Black American youth. The opiate crisis has continuously pushed them into devastation and crisis of incarceration, separating them from the rest of family members. Besides, there were wars on drug use policies that are misused by the law enforcement authorities, who target Black neighbourhoods.

Consequently, the number of Blacks dying from opioid has reached an extended rate higher than the general population in numerous states such as Missouri, Illinois, Minnesota, Wisconsin, West Virginia and Washington, D.C. For example, these rates in the States of Virginia and Wisconsin have the number of Blacks with fatal overdose nearly double that of Caucasian. The discussion provides more data in Chicago and Illinois which are the most affected cities. Despite making up to 15% of the Illinois population, Blacks account for about one-quarter of opioid overdose deaths.

On the other hand, Chicago alone has had an extreme increase in a fatal opioid overdose that rose up to 75%. Besides, Chicago has got approximately 32% of the population made of Black people but they account for about half of all opioid deaths which are 48.4%. Moreover, in 2016 Chicago that rate of Blacks' deaths was 56% which was higher than the white death rate from opioids. Consequently, the CDC data reveals that African American deaths in Chicago in 2016 were almost four times more elevated than the national average rate in 2015.

References

1. American Addiction Centers. Race and Addiction. 2018.

2. Johnson RS. The racial divide in the opioid epidemic. Modern Healthcare. 2016.

3. Volkow ND and McLellan TA. Opioid Abuse in Chronic Pain-Misconceptions and Mitigation Strategies. N Engl J Med. 2016; 374: 1253-1263.

4. Confronting the Opioid crisis in the United States. Opioids.gov. 2018.

5. Cheng HG and Phillips MR. Secondary analysis of existing data: opportunities and implementation. Shanghai Archives of Psychiatry. 2014; 26: 371-375.

6. Bechteler SS and Kane-Willis K. The African American Opioid Epidemic. Chicago Urban League. 2017.

7. Squires LE, Palfai TP, Allensworth-Davies D, Cheng DM, Bernstein J, et al. Perceived discrimination, racial identity, and health behaviors among black primary-care patients who use drugs. J Ethn Subst Abuse. 2017; 1-18.

8. Chicago department of public health. Epidemiology report: Increase in overdose deaths involving opioids-Chicago, 2015-2016. 2017.

9. Hansen H and Netherland J. Is the Prescription Opioid Epidemic a White Problem? American Journal of Public Health. 2016; 106: 2127-2129.

10. Escamilla J and Gatens A. Illinois opioid Prescription data. Criminal Justice data. 2018.

11. Roster of commissioners. The president's commission on combating drug addiction and the Opioid crisis. Whitehouse.gov. 2017.

12. Peteet BJ. Psychosocial risks of prescription drug misuse among U.S. racial/ethnic minorities: A systematic review. J Ethn Subst Abuse. 2017; 1-33.

> *"The researchers hypothesized that men and women would be affected by overdose deaths at the same rates."*

Men Are at Higher Risk of Overdosing on Opioids

Brown University

Overdose deaths spiked across the U.S. during the COVID-19 pandemic, but some groups were affected more than others, according to a study by researchers at Brown University's School of Public Health. These groups include people experiencing joblessness, people who used synthetic opioids, and men. Men made up the vast majority of overdoses in the study, accounting for 77 percent of them. Some of the effects of the pandemic—including an unstable job market, lost wages, and mental health issues—contributed to an increase in overdoses, but more research must be done on why men especially experienced this spike. Brown University is a research university in Providence, Rhode Island.

As you read, consider the following questions:

1. According to this viewpoint, which groups of people experienced the highest rates of overdoses during the COVID-19 pandemic?

"Men, Jobless and People with Mental Health Diagnoses Most Vulnerable in 2020 Overdose Spike," Brown University, September 17, 2021. Reprinted by permission.

2. What changes that occurred during the pandemic contributed to changes in overdose rates, as described in this viewpoint?

3. Are the researchers mentioned in this viewpoint able to explain why men experienced a higher overdose death rate than women?

At the same time as COVID-19 has claimed more than 600,000 lives across the United States, drug overdose deaths across the nation reached unprecedented heights. Rhode Island has been particularly affected: In December 2020, the state had the highest rate in the country of COVID-19 cases and deaths relevant to population; during the first eight months of 2020, the rate of unintentional drug overdose deaths in Rhode Island increased 28% relative to the same period in the prior year.

Researchers at Brown University's School of Public Health wanted to learn more about the causes of the overdoses during the pandemic, as well as the people affected by them, as scant data were available. They analyzed two years of health data to look for trends and patterns.

According to their study, published on Friday, Sept. 17, in JAMA Network Open, men, individuals who had lost jobs and people with mental health diagnoses experienced the largest increases in rates of overdose deaths during the pandemic. The researchers also found increases in deaths involving synthetic opioids and in deaths occurring in personal residences (compared to a hospital or elsewhere).

"Our motivation for this study was to understand more about the causes and characteristics of these overdose deaths and to identify some of the groups of people who are at heightened risk of overdose during the pandemic," said Alexandria Macmadu, a study co-author and Ph.D. candidate in epidemiology at Brown.

The team analyzed information from four statewide databases linked via the Rhode Island Data Ecosystem. They compared the characteristics of 264 adults in the state who died from an overdose during the first eight months of 2020 to those of 206 adults who died from an overdose during the same period in the year prior, examining variables such as age, sex, race and ethnicity, as well as the type of drug contributing to death, location of death and socioeconomic factors such as housing insecurity, job loss and wages.

"These linked statewide databases really allowed us to take a deeper dive into this topic," Macmadu said. "For example, by using data from the state Department of Labor and Training, we were able to correlate overdose deaths and recent job loss; using Medicaid data, we were able to correlate overdose deaths with mental health diagnosis, to the level that we could identify, say, people in their 50s with anxiety as having elevated risk."

The findings show that overdoses increased significantly among males (who accounted for 72% of deaths in 2019 vs. 77% in 2020), people using synthetic opioids (71% vs. 76%) and occurring in personal residences (45% vs. 53%). People experiencing job loss represented a greater portion of overdose deaths (who accounted for 8% of deaths in 2019 vs. 16% in 2020), and there was an increase in overdoses in subgroups of people with mental health diagnoses.

The researchers hypothesized that men and women would be affected by overdose deaths at the same rates, said Brandon Marshall, study corresponding author and an associate professor of epidemiology at Brown's School of Public Health.

"To see the significant increase in overdose deaths among men was surprising," Marshall said. "I don't think we have a good explanation for that at this time, and it's something that requires further research."

The researchers note that differences between overdose deaths in 2020 compared to 2019 correspond to changes that occurred during the pandemic, including increased isolation, an onslaught of mental health stressors, widespread economic insecurity and the lethality of the drug supply. The new findings provide guidance for clinicians, public health officials, scientists, policymakers and others who hope to stem the tide of overdose deaths, the researchers said.

As an example, they cite the finding that a significant number of people were pronounced dead from an overdose in their personal residence.

"We already know that many people were socially and physically isolated during the early months of the pandemic," Marshall said. "Our findings show that, as a result of the pandemic, a significant number of people are using drugs alone right now — which means there's no bystander available to intervene or call 911. This greatly increases overdose risk."

The researchers offer a number of recommendations to address this risk, including the strengthening of Good Samaritan law protections for those who call 911; state establishment of pilot harm reduction centers to provide a safer, supervised environment for drug use; and safely prioritizing in-person recovery services to enhance support for socially isolated individuals at high risk of overdose.

These recommendations for interventions to reduce overdose deaths will still be highly applicable to a post-pandemic world, Macmadu said. In fact, some of the changes that have been made in response to the pandemic, including audio-only telehealth consultations to begin addiction treatment with buprenorphine, will be highly beneficial even when the world opens up and returns to a new normal.

The authors said it's notable and timely that Rhode Island recently became the first state to authorize overdose prevention sites, or "harm reduction centers" — places where people can safely use drugs under medical supervision, and where trained staff can connect them to evidence-based harm reduction strategies and programs. Creating these sites is a step in the right direction in battling the opioid epidemic, they said.

"Continued expansion of access to evidence-based treatment and harm reduction programs for people who use drugs will be critical in addressing the epidemic of overdose deaths, during a viral pandemic as well as in the future," Macmadu said.

"America must deal with our pain epidemic if we have any hope of dealing with the painkiller epidemic."

Understanding Why Some Groups Are Hit Harder Than Others Could Curb Opioid Addiction

Susan Sered

In the following viewpoint Susan Sered argues in favor of more research that studies why some demographic groups are more affected by the opioid crisis than others. While the US government aims to address the opioid crisis through treatment of addiction, it is equally important to understand the root causes of the crisis. Identifying how particular groups deal with their unique pain can lay the groundwork for prevention. Susan Sered is a medical sociologist, Professor of Sociology at Suffolk University and author of Can't Catch a Break: Gender, Jail, Drugs, and the Limits of Personal Responsibility.

As you read, consider the following questions:

1. What is "primary prevention," according to the author?
2. How can social science address issues with the opioid problem that medical science does not?

"How Understanding Pain Could Curb Opioid Addiction," by Susan Sered, The Conversation, May 15, 2018, https://theconversation.com/how-understanding-pain-could-curb-opioid-addiction-95995. Licensed under CC BY-ND 4.0.

3. For which demographic did the opioid-related overdose rate triple in Massachusetts, according to the viewpoint?

The Senate Health, Education, Labor and Pensions Committee unanimously approved a bill in April 2018 designed to address the opioid crisis. The bill called the Opioid Crisis Response Act of 2018 covers much of the same territory as the 138-page report released in November 2017 by a commission appointed by President Donald Trump.

Both the Senate bill and the commission document, unlike the president's own March 2018 call for executing drug dealers, recognize addiction as a health problem and focus on treatment rather than punishment.

All of this is important, but as a medical sociologist, I am particularly interested in developing better understandings of the root causes of the current crisis. Why are so many Americans willing to ingest substances that, they most likely know, can lead to grievous harm? In other words, I am interested in the demand side of opioid overuse.

A Little Prevention, but How Much Cure?

For prevention, the Senate bill calls for expanding prescription monitoring programs, amping up the ability to seize illegal drugs at U.S. borders, training health care providers in proper prescribing practices, and improving drug disposal systems. All of these measures are what we sociologists consider "secondary prevention"; that is, they are directed toward supply reduction.

Primary prevention—which deals with the reasons that people turn to opioids in the first place—is mentioned in the Senate bill in only a few places but is not developed either in terms of a research plan nor in terms of public health strategies. The president's commission report briefly deals with prevention in terms of school and media programs designed to inform children and parents about the dangers of opioid use.

In my experience, this does not address many of the issues that lead people to opioids. The Massachusetts women with whom I have been conducting research for the past decade began their substance abuse careers in pain, either mental or physical. In some cases, the pain was a consequence of childhood or intimate partner abuse. In other cases, the pain set in because underlying health problems were not attended to properly or in a timely manner.

Often, the pain wasn't taken seriously by employers, who insisted that minimum wage workers show up even when they are unwell, family members or health care providers. While substantive help often wasn't available, psychotropic and pain medication was easy to get hold of, whether from doctors or drug dealers or both.

Following these women in and out of drug treatment for years, I have come to think that America must deal with our pain epidemic if we have any hope of dealing with the painkiller epidemic.

Though it is only a brief reference, it is heartening that the Senate bill calls upon the NIH "to improve scientific understanding of pain, including how to prevent, treat, and manage pain."

Medical science primarily focuses on the physiological and neurological pathways associated with pain in the individual body. Social science pays more attention to pain in the "social body"—in the environmental, economic, political and cultural conditions that give rise to collective experiences of suffering, hopelessness or exclusion. The social science approach is particularly appropriate in the case of a crisis that, at least to some observers, has reached "epidemic" proportions.

Gender, Race and Class

The Senate bill acknowledges that not all states have been equally affected by the opioid crisis, but it does not explicitly call for research into why particular communities and demographic groups are harder hit than others.

Data indicate that opioid abuse is primarily a male problem, concentrated in working class and low-income white communities, and rapidly expanding to Hispanic communities. That does not mean that women or professional class Americans are not affected by opioid overuse. It does mean that particular groups seem to have developed particularly fertile ground for opioid misuse to take root.

According to a Massachusetts report on opiate-related hospital discharges by ZIP code, low-income and working-class neighborhoods have substantially higher rates of opioid problems than upper-middle-class neighborhoods. Department of Public Health data for the state also show a pronounced gender difference in death rates from opioid-related causes: Men are four times more likely than women to die from opioids. And while the current opioid crisis tends to be described a problem of white communities, in Massachusetts the opioid-related overdose death rate for Hispanics tripled from 2014 to 2016.

Information of this sort lays the groundwork for primary prevention. What is it about being male in a white low-income community that causes pain and makes opioid use attractive as a means of dealing with pain? Are there occupational or educational policies that encourage or discourage substance abuse? And can those policies be adjusted in ways that reduce pain as well as substance abuse?

Recent preliminary research points to a number of directions that may be useful in terms of getting at root causes. I am particularly interested in several quantitative and qualitative studies that link low social capital, social isolation, weak community ties and economic despair to higher opioid abuse rates. Overall, however, considering the extent of the opioid crisis, there is surprisingly little written addressing root causes. It will be interesting to track the outcomes of projects such as the San Francisco initiative to train low-income and formerly incarcerated women as birth doulas or the Boston area Haley House that includes formerly incarcerated men in community kitchen and garden enterprises.

Regardless of what proposals become official policy, I believe that better understanding why people turn to opioids in the first place can be an important part of our national response.

Periodical and Internet Sources Bibliography

The following articles have been selected to supplement the diverse views presented in this chapter.

Richard Florida, "The Changing Geography of the Opioid Crisis," *Bloomberg CityLab,* December 5, 2019. https://www.bloomberg. com/news/articles/2019-12-05/how-opioid-deaths-differ-in-rural-and-urban-areas.

Jon Kamp and Julie Wernau, "Opioid Overdose Death Rate for U.S. Black Population Is Higher Than for White," *Wall Street Journal,* March 13, 2022. https://www.wsj.com/articles/opioid-overdose-death-rate-for-u-s-black-population-is-higher-than-for-white-11647176400.

Maryann Mason, Rebekah Soliman, and Howard S. Kim, "Disparities by Sex and Race and Ethnicity in Death Rates Due to Opioid Overdose Among Adults 55 Years and Older, 1999 to 2019," *JAMA Network Open*, January 11, 2022. https://jamanetwork. com/journals/jamanetworkopen/fullarticle/2787930.

David Powell, "Understanding the Demographics of the Opioid Overdose Death Crisis," RAND Corporation, October 2021. https://www.rand.org/content/dam/rand/pubs/working_papers/ WRA1400/WRA1484-2/RAND_WRA1484-2.pdf.

Steven Reinberg, "U.S. Opioid ODs Cluster in Centers of Poverty," *HealthDay*, March 26, 2018. https://consumer.healthday.com/ bone-and-joint-information-4/opioids-990/u-s-opioid-ods-cluster-in-centers-of-poverty-732258.html.

Mary-Russell Roberson, "Tracking the Shifting Landscape of the Opioid Crisis," *Tufts Now*, September 21, 2021. https://now.tufts. edu/articles/tracking-shifting-landscape-opioid-crisis.

Steven Ross Johnson, "Study: Opioid Deaths Have Surged Among Older Black Men," *US News & World Report*, January 11, 2022. https://www.usnews.com/news/health-news/articles/2022-01-11/ study-opioid-deaths-have-surged-among-older-black-men.

Susan Salmond and Virginia Allread, "A Population Health Approach to America's Opioid Epidemic," *Orthopedic Nursing*, March/April 2019. https://journals.lww.com/orthopaedicnursing/Fulltext/2019/03000/A_Population_Health_Approach_to_America_s_Opioid.4.aspx.

Shanoor Seervai, Arnav Shah, and Eric C. Schneider, "The US Has Two Opioid Epidemics: The Federal Response Should Consider Both," the Commonwealth Fund, March 22, 2018. https://www.commonwealthfund.org/blog/2018/us-has-two-opioid-epidemics-federal-response-should-consider-both.

Abdullah Shihipar, "Opinion: The Opioid Crisis Isn't White," *New York Times*, February 26, 2019. https://www.nytimes.com/2019/02/26/opinion/opioid-crisis-drug-users.html.

Ahlishia Shipley, "Opioid Crisis Affects All Americans, Rural and Urban," US Department of Agriculture (USDA), August 3, 2021. https://www.usda.gov/media/blog/2018/01/11/opioid-crisis-affects-all-americans-rural-and-urban.

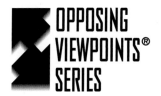

OPPOSING
VIEWPOINTS®
SERIES

CHAPTER 3

Who Is Responsible for the Opioid Crisis, and Can They Be Held Accountable?

Chapter Preface

Responsibility for the opioid crisis is a challenging topic. The American public and many experts—including those in law enforcement, the justice system, politics, and journalism—would like a simple answer regarding who is to blame. In many ways, the Purdue Pharma pharmaceutical company and its owners, the Sacklers, have served as an acceptable answer to this question, and numerous experts agree that they deserve to bear responsibility. However, it has proven difficult to determine how best to legally hold them accountable and what can be accomplished with such accountability.

Since approximately 2007, Purdue Pharma has faced an overwhelming number of lawsuits filed on behalf of individuals affected by prescription opioid abuse and also on behalf of U.S. states. By September 2019, up against a total of approximately 3,000 lawsuits, Purdue Pharma filed for bankruptcy.[1] The terms of the bankruptcy settlements have repeatedly faced opposition from states and lawyers. This is because although the terms of the settlement would involve the Sackler family paying billions of dollars to be used for opioid treatment, research, and support for victims, the family has also insisted that the settlement would release the family from any current or future lawsuits.[2] While under these terms Purdue Pharma would cease to exist, the Sacklers would no longer be allowed to produce or sell opioids, and the family would be forced to pay billions of dollars to help undo the damage, shielding the family from lawsuits filed by victims of the opioid crisis strikes many Americans as unjust. Consequently, as of early 2022, the struggle to sort out accountability for Purdue Pharma and the Sacklers continues in court.

During the 2022 bankruptcy hearing, individuals who had been harmed by the drug OxyContin were allowed to confront members of the Sackler family for the first time. Over two hours, approximately two dozen people described the pain Purdue

Pharma had inflicted on their families to three members of the Sackler family.[3] The Sacklers did not respond to these statements or offer an apology, but the fact that they were confronted face-to-face by those they had harmed offered some amount of catharsis.

However, for many, the downfall of Purdue Pharma and the Sackler family does not entirely resolve the question of blame. This is because various experts agree that Purdue Pharma could not have caused the opioid crisis on its own. The company needed doctors and health-care providers to prescribe its opioids on a massive scale, federal government agencies like the Food and Drug Administration (FDA) and the Drug Enforcement Administration (DEA) to allow its drugs to be widely prescribed and distributed, and pharmacies to willingly fill these prescriptions. Furthermore, the company needed the American public to be willing to take its medications, and to keep on taking them. For this reason, experts in this chapter argue that many others deserve scrutiny for their roles in the opioid crisis as well.

This chapter will look at how Purdue Pharma and the Sacklers have faced accountability for the opioid crisis while also examining the issue of responsibility through a broader lens to consider who else has played a role in this disturbing era in American history.

Notes

1. Brendan Pierson, Mike Spector, and Maria Chutchian, "US Judge Tosses $4.5 Bln Deal Shielding Sacklers from Opioid Lawsuits," Reuters, December 16, 2021. https://www.reuters.com/business/judge-tosses-deal-shielding-purdues-sackler-family-opioid-claims-2021-12-17/.
2. *Ibid.*
3. Guardian Staff and Agencies, "Sacklers Confronted by Opioid Crisis Victims and Families at Virtual Hearing," the *Guardian,* March 10, 2022. https://www.theguardian.com/us-news/2022/mar/10/sacklers-opioid-crisis-victims-families-hearing/.

> *"Purdue Pharma actively thwarted the United States' efforts to ensure compliance and prevent diversion. The devastating ripple effect of Purdue's actions left lives lost and others addicted."*

The U.S. Federal Government Has Led Civil and Criminal Investigations into the Opioid Crisis

United States Department of Justice

After years of investigations by numerous US federal agencies, including the Federal Bureau of Investigation (FBI) and the Drug Enforcement Administration (DEA), the US Department of Justice resolved criminal and civil investigations into the Purdue Pharma pharmaceutical company in October 2020. It also resolved civil claims against the Sackler family, the company's owners, though they did not face any criminal charges. The settlement would cost the company at least $8 billion and the Sackler family $225 million. These investigations allowed for greater transparency into Purdue Pharma's misdeeds and led to some amount of legal accountability. The US Department of Justice is the department of the federal government responsible for enforcing federal law and administering justice.

"Justice Department Announces Global Resolution of Criminal and Civil Investigations with Opioid Manufacturer Purdue Pharma and Civil Settlement with Members of the Sackler Family," The United States Department of Justice, October 21, 2020. Reprinted by permission.

As you read, consider the following questions:

1. What did Purdue Pharma admit to doing as part of their criminal plea?
2. How much will the Sackler family pay in damages because of their False Claims Act liability?
3. What is one important condition to the resolution of Purdue Pharma's criminal and civil investigations, according to this viewpoint?

Today, the Department of Justice announced a global resolution of its criminal and civil investigations into the opioid manufacturer Purdue Pharma LP (Purdue), and a civil resolution of its civil investigation into individual shareholders from the Sackler family. The resolutions with Purdue are subject to the approval of the bankruptcy court.

"The abuse and diversion of prescription opioids has contributed to a national tragedy of addiction and deaths, in addition to those caused by illicit street opioids," said Deputy Attorney General Jeffrey A. Rosen. "With criminal guilty pleas, a federal settlement of more than $8 billion, and the dissolution of a company and repurposing its assets entirely for the public's benefit, the resolution in today's announcement re-affirms that the Department of Justice will not relent in its multi-pronged efforts to combat the opioids crisis."

"Today's resolution is the result of years of hard work by the FBI and its partners to combat the opioid crisis in the U.S.," said Steven M. D'Antuono, Assistant Director in Charge of the FBI Washington Field Office. "Purdue, through greed and violation of the law, prioritized money over the health and well-being of patients. The FBI remains committed to holding companies accountable for their illegal and inexcusable activity and to seeking justice, on behalf of the victims, for those who contributed to the opioid crisis."

"The opioid epidemic remains a significant public health challenge that impacts the lives of men and women across the country," said Gary L. Cantrell Deputy Inspector General for Investigations at the U.S. Department of Health and Human Services' Office of Inspector General. "Unfortunately, Purdue's reckless actions and violation of the law senselessly risked patients' health and well-being. With our law enforcement partners, we will continue to combat the opioid crisis, including holding the pharmaceutical industry and its executives accountable."

"This resolution closes a particularly sad chapter in the ongoing battle against opioid addiction," said Drug Enforcement Administration (DEA) Assistant Administrator Tim McDermott. "Purdue Pharma actively thwarted the United States' efforts to ensure compliance and prevent diversion. The devastating ripple effect of Purdue's actions left lives lost and others addicted. DEA will continue to work tirelessly with our partners and the pharmaceutical industry to address the damage that has been done, and bring an end to this epidemic that has gripped the nation for far too long."

Purdue Pharma has agreed to plead guilty in federal court in New Jersey to a three-count felony information charging it with one count of dual-object conspiracy to defraud the United States and to violate the Food, Drug, and Cosmetic Act, and two counts of conspiracy to violate the Federal Anti-Kickback Statute. The criminal resolution includes the largest penalties ever levied against a pharmaceutical manufacturer, including a criminal fine of $3.544 billion and an additional $2 billion in criminal forfeiture. For the $2 billion forfeiture, the company will pay $225 million on the effective date of the bankruptcy, and, as further explained below, the department is willing to credit the value conferred by the company to State and local governments under the department's anti-piling on and coordination policy. Purdue has also agreed to a civil settlement in the amount of $2.8 billion to resolve its civil liability under the False Claims Act. Separately, the Sackler family has agreed to pay $225 million in damages to resolve its civil False Claims Act liability.

The resolutions do not include the criminal release of any individuals, including members of the Sackler family, nor are any of the company's executives or employees receiving civil releases.

While the global resolution with the company is subject to approval by the bankruptcy court in the Southern District of New York, one important condition in the resolution is that the company would cease to operate in its current form and would instead emerge from bankruptcy as a public benefit company (PBC) owned by a trust or similar entity designed for the benefit of the American public, to function entirely in the public interest. Indeed, not only will the PBC endeavor to deliver legitimate prescription drugs in a manner as safe as possible, but it will aim to donate, or provide steep discounts for, life-saving overdose rescue drugs and medically assisted treatment medications to communities, and the proceeds of the trust will be directed toward State and local opioid abatement programs. Based on the value that would be conferred to State and local governments through the PBC, the department is willing to credit up to $1.775 billion against the agreed $2 billion forfeiture amount. The department looks forward to working with the creditor groups in the bankruptcy in charting the path forward for this PBC so that its public health goals can be best accomplished.

The Criminal Pleas

As part of the plea, Purdue will admit that from May 2007 through at least March 2017, Purdue conspired to defraud the United States by impeding the lawful function of the DEA by representing to the DEA that Purdue maintained an effective anti-diversion program when, in fact, Purdue continued to market its opioid products to more than 100 health care providers whom the company had good reason to believe were diverting opioids and by reporting misleading information to the DEA to boost Purdue's manufacturing quotas. The misleading information comprised prescription data that included prescriptions written by doctors that Purdue had good reason to believe were engaged in diversion. The conspiracy also involved aiding and abetting violations of the Food, Drug, and Cosmetic Act by facilitating the dispensing of its opioid products, including OxyContin, without a legitimate medical purpose, and thus without lawful prescriptions.

In addition, Purdue will admit to conspiring to violate the Federal Anti-Kickback Statute. Between June 2009 and March 2017, Purdue made payments to two doctors through Purdue's doctor speaker program to induce those doctors to write more prescriptions of Purdue's opioid products. Similarly, from approximately April 2016 through December 2016, Purdue made payments to Practice Fusion Inc., an electronic health records company, in exchange for referring, recommending, and arranging for the ordering of Purdue's extended release opioid products—OxyContin, Butrans, and Hysingla.

The Civil Settlements

The department's civil settlements resolve the United States' claims as to both Purdue and its individual shareholders, members of the Sackler family.

The civil settlement with Purdue provides the United States with an allowed, unsubordinated, general unsecured bankruptcy claim for recovery of $2.8 billion. This settlement resolves allegations that from 2010 to 2018, Purdue caused false claims to be submitted to federal health care programs, specifically Medicare, Medicaid, TRICARE, the Federal Employees Health Benefits Program, and the Indian Health Service. The government alleged that Purdue promoted its opioid drugs to health care providers it knew were prescribing opioids for uses that were unsafe, ineffective, and medically unnecessary, and that often led to abuse and diversion. For example, Purdue learned that one doctor was known by patients as "the Candyman" and was prescribing "crazy dosing of OxyContin," yet Purdue had sales representatives meet with the doctor more than 300 times. It also resolves the government's allegations that Purdue engaged in three different kickback schemes to induce prescriptions of its opioids. First, Purdue paid certain doctors ostensibly to provide educational talks to other health care professionals and serve as consultants, but in reality to induce them to prescribe more OxyContin. Second, Purdue paid kickbacks to Practice Fusion, as described above. Third, Purdue entered into contracts with certain specialty pharmacies to fill prescriptions for Purdue's opioid drugs that other pharmacies had rejected as potentially lacking medical necessity.

Under a separate civil settlement, individual members of the Sackler family will pay the United States $225 million arising from the alleged conduct of Dr. Richard Sackler, David Sackler, Mortimer D.A. Sackler, Dr. Kathe Sackler, and Jonathan Sackler (the Named Sacklers). This settlement resolves allegations that, in 2012, the Named Sacklers knew that the legitimate market for Purdue's opioids had contracted. Nevertheless, they requested that Purdue executives recapture lost sales and increase Purdue's share of the opioid market. The Named Sacklers then approved a new marketing program beginning in 2013 called "Evolve to Excellence," through which Purdue sales representatives intensified their marketing of OxyContin to extreme, high-volume prescribers who were already writing "25 times as many OxyContin scripts" as their peers, causing health care providers to prescribe opioids for uses that were unsafe, ineffective, and medically unnecessary, and that often led to abuse and diversion.

The civil settlement also resolves the government's allegations that from approximately 2008 to 2018, at the Named Sacklers' request, Purdue transferred assets into Sackler family holding companies and trusts that were made to hinder future creditors, and/or were otherwise voidable as fraudulent transfers.

Today's resolution does not resolve claims that states may have against Purdue or members of the Sackler family, nor does it impede the debtors' ability to recover any fraudulent transfers.

Today's announcement was made by Deputy Attorney General Jeffrey A. Rosen; Acting Assistant Attorney General of the Civil

Division Jeffrey Clark; U.S. Attorney for the District of Vermont Christina Nolan; and First Assistant U.S. Attorney for the District of New Jersey Rachael Honig. The criminal investigation was conducted by the U.S. Attorney's Offices for the Districts of New Jersey and Vermont, the Consumer Protection Branch of the Department of Justice's Civil Division, and the FBI's Washington, D.C. and Newark Field Offices, with assistance by the DEA and the U.S. Attorney's Office for the Northern District of Ohio. The civil settlements were handled by the Fraud Section of the Commercial Litigation Branch of the Department of Justice's Civil Division, and the U.S. Attorney's Offices for the Districts of New Jersey and Vermont, with assistance from the Department of Health and Human Services, Office of General Counsel and Office of Counsel to the Inspector General; the Defense Health Agency; and the Office of Personnel Management. The Purdue bankruptcy matter is being handled by the U.S. Attorney's Office for the Southern District of New York and the Civil Division's Commercial Litigation Branch, Corporate/Finance Section.

Except to the extent of Purdue's admissions as part of its criminal resolution, the claims resolved by the civil settlements are allegations only. There has been no determination of liability in the civil matters.

> "The crackdown on legally produced
> opioids has driven nonmedical users
> toward black-market substitutes
> that are far more dangerous
> because their potency is inconsistent
> and unpredictable."

The U.S. Government Is Also Responsible for the Opioid Crisis

Jacob Sullum

Although many have blamed pharmaceutical companies like Purdue Pharma for causing the opioid crisis, Jacob Sullum argues that the U.S. federal government shares some of the responsibility for it. The Food and Drug Administration (FDA) approved the opioid drugs that people became addicted to, which suggests that they failed to protect the American public. The Drug Enforcement Administration (DEA) also did little in response to the fact that opioid overdose deaths surged. The Center for Disease Control and Prevention (CDC) issued guidelines that led to drastic dose reductions. This viewpoint argues that while pharmaceutical companies may have helped start the opioid crisis, the federal government, and to some extent medical professionals, allowed it to get out of hand. Jacob Sullum is a senior editor at Reason and a nationally syndicated columnist.

"Should We Blame Pharmacies or the Government for Opioid-Related Deaths?" by Jacob Sullum, Reason.com and Reason magazine, November 24, 2021. Reprinted by permission.

As you read, consider the following questions:

1. Aside from legal drug suppliers, what are some of the links in the long causal chain of opioid-related addiction and deaths?
2. Why would doctors comply with the new CDC guidelines even if they knew they were inappropriate?
3. What explains the drastic increase in opioid-related deaths after the prescribing rate had fallen by almost half?

A federal jury in Cleveland yesterday concluded that three major pharmacy chains had contributed to a "public nuisance" in two Ohio counties caused by an oversupply of prescription opioids. The verdict, which represents the first time that retailers have been held legally liable for the "opioid crisis," followed two recent rulings in which a California judge and the Oklahoma Supreme Court rejected similar claims against drug manufacturers.

These cases, along with thousands of other lawsuits by state and local governments that blame legal drug suppliers for opioid-related addiction and deaths, ask courts to focus on one link in a long causal chain. That chain includes decisions by state and federal regulators as well as actions by manufacturers, distributors, doctors, pharmacists, patients, black-market dealers who sell diverted pills, and nonmedical users who consume them.

In the Ohio case, Lake and Trumbull counties argued that the defendants—CVS, Walgreens, and Walmart—had ignored "red flags" indicating that some of the prescriptions they filled were medically inappropriate. The defendants argued that they had done nothing but fill seemingly legitimate prescriptions for legally approved medication written by licensed and regulated doctors. They emphasized the crucial roles that government agencies such as the Food and Drug Administration (FDA) and the Drug Enforcement Administration played in overseeing the distribution of prescription opioids, making them complicit in the supposed public nuisance described by the plaintiffs.

The government is likewise responsible for the harm caused by its ham-handed efforts to reduce opioid prescriptions, as illustrated by a recent case involving a Kentucky man, Brent Slone, who killed himself after his pain medication was suddenly slashed. His wife, CaSonya Richardson-Slone, sued Commonwealth Pain and Spine, which operated the clinic she blamed for denying her husband proper pain treatment. Last August, a Louisville jury awarded her and the couple's daughter $7 million in damages. As STAT reporter Andrew Joseph's thorough and illuminating account of the case shows, the situation that drove Slone to suicide is a predictable result of the government's demonstrably counterproductive attempt to reduce opioid-related deaths by limiting access to pain medication.

In a 2011 car crash, Joseph reports, Slone suffered "a broken pelvis, a compressed spinal cord, and other injuries that caused chronic pain and put him in a wheelchair." He was already taking opioids for pain relief in 2014, when he sought treatment at Commonwealth Pain and Spine. His daily dosage at the time was about 240 morphine milligram equivalents (MME), but it would eventually rise to a peak of 540 MME after a series of surgeries.

As Joseph notes, Slone's treatment "coincided with campaigns to rectify opioid prescribing." Responding to rising opioid-related deaths, regulators and legislators sought to discourage pain pill prescriptions across the board. In the effort to drive down consumption of opioid analgesics, chronic pain patients like Slone, who account for a disproportionate share of the total, were an obvious target.

Between 2010 and 2017, the number of opioid prescriptions per 100 Americans fell by 28 percent. During the same period, the rate of high-dose opioid prescriptions—defined as 90 MME or more per day—fell by 56 percent. In 2016, the Centers for Disease Control and Prevention (CDC) further encouraged the latter trend by publishing guidelines that were widely interpreted (misinterpreted, according to the CDC) as recommending that doctors stay below the arbitrary 90-MME cutoff.

Given the tremendous pressure on doctors to curtail the use of opioid analgesics, it would be surprising if all the dose reductions resulting from "campaigns to rectify opioid prescribing" were medically appropriate. Doctors had good reason to worry that they were risking their licenses and livelihoods if they defied the new conventional wisdom by maintaining patients on high doses of opioids, even if they had been taking them for years and the benefits seemed to outweigh the risks. Complaints about the consequences of the CDC's guidelines, which included many reports of abrupt and drastic cutbacks in medication as well as outright denial of treatment, suggested that more than a few doctors sacrificed patient welfare to avoid unwanted attention.

While the benefits of long-term, high-dose opioid therapy are a contentious subject, Joseph notes, "experts and governmental guidelines agree that—with few exceptions—dose reductions need to go slowly, with patient buy-in." But that is not what happened with Slone.

In 2016, the same year the CDC issued its controversial advice, Slone "started traveling to California for advanced wound care," because his wheelchair had "caused pressure sores that resulted in bone infections." After a series of surgeries that included skin grafts, Slone spent several weeks at a nursing facility in La Jolla, and "his daily opioid intake increased from 240 MME to above 400 MME, occasionally reaching 540 MME." He was discharged with a prescription at the latter level.

When Slone returned to Kentucky, one of his doctors at the pain clinic initially wrote him a 540 MME per day "bridge" prescription. But at an appointment about a week later, Slone's dosage was suddenly reduced by 56 percent, to 240 MME per day. Exactly why that happened is a matter of dispute.

"The defense framed Slone's reduction as intentional," Joseph writes. "The higher dose of 540 MME reflected what Slone was on for acute pain following surgery, at a time when he was closely monitored at inpatient facilities. Such a dose would not be safe for him out in the world. They were simply moving him back to his chronic pain baseline dose, and claimed he would not experience withdrawal because 240 MME was still supplying a sufficient opioid amount."

By contrast, Hans Poppe, Richardson-Slone's lawyer, "pointed to testimony indicating that a nurse inadvertently slashed Slone's dose to his prior one—perhaps because she copied over information from his chart from months earlier—and that the doctors didn't catch the error." At the trial, Poppe described the change as a clear case of "patient abandonment," and the jury evidently agreed.

Whether the sharp drop in Slone's dosage was deliberate or accidental, it certainly seems inconsistent with recommendations that doctors who decide to "taper" patients begin with a reduction of about 10 percent. "This is the problem that we see," Beth Darnall, a psychologist who directs the Stanford Pain Relief Innovations Lab, told Joseph. "There is this rush, almost a panic, to decrease doses rapidly under the guise of patient safety, but the irony is these rapid changes expose patients to greater risk."

Stefan Kertesz, a University of Alabama at Birmingham pain and addiction specialist, agreed "it was a dose change that people would not be expected to tolerate." It is fair to say that Slone, who killed himself a few weeks after his dose was cut, did not find it tolerable.

Kertesz, who is researching suicides following abrupt tapering, helped organize a 2019 letter from hundreds of experts who were alarmed by the practice. In response, then–CDC Director Robert Redfield emphasized that the agency "does not endorse mandated or abrupt dose reduction or discontinuation, as these actions can result in patient harm." He said the CDC recommends that clinicians "work with patients to taper or reduce dosage only when patient harm outweighs patient benefit of opioid therapy." It "also recommends that the plan be based on the patient's goals and concerns and that tapering be slow enough to minimize opioid withdrawal, e.g., 10 percent a week or 10 percent a month for patients who have been on high-dose opioids for years."

In a "safety announcement" issued the same day, the FDA said it had "received reports of serious harm in patients who are physically dependent on opioid pain medicines suddenly having these medicines discontinued or the dose rapidly decreased." It warned that the consequences "include serious withdrawal symptoms, uncontrolled pain, psychological distress, and suicide."

The CDC is in the process of revising its opioid prescribing advice. "Some policies and practices citing the guideline went beyond its recommendations and were inconsistent with its guidance," Deborah Dowell, who co-authored the guidelines, said at a meeting in July. "For example, the guideline does not support abrupt tapering or sudden discontinuation of opioids, but we heard many reports of it being inappropriately cited to justify suddenly cutting off opioids."

The harm to patients is not the only cost of restrictions on pain medication. As of last year, the overall opioid prescribing rate had fallen by 48 percent since 2012. During the same period, opioid-related deaths more than tripled. Last year about 83 percent of those deaths involved illicit fentanyl.

"U.S. opioid prescribing has plummeted in the past decade," Joseph notes, "even as the overdose crisis has reached record heights due to an explosion of illicit fentanyl." That is hardly a coincidence, since the crackdown on legally produced opioids has driven nonmedical users toward black-market substitutes that are far more dangerous because their potency is inconsistent and unpredictable.

Which brings us back to the lawsuit against CVS, Walgreens, and Walmart. To make their case, the counties that sued the pharmacy chains had to show that the public nuisance they alleged was ongoing. "The counties' lawyers successfully argued that when the supply receded, patients who were addicted to the pills had turned to heroin and illegal fentanyl," The New York Times reports. "That result was a foreseeable, direct descendant of the floods of prescription opioid pills, the lawyers said."

It is a mistake to describe all of those opioid users as "patients," which implies that the drugs typically were prescribed for them and that they became addicted as a result of pain treatment, something that happens much less often than commonly thought. But the Times is right that restricting the supply of legally produced opioids had predictably lethal effects.

> *"Unscrupulous 'pill mill' doctors could have a big effect on the painkiller supply in some states, CDC researchers argued, pointing to a 2011 study ... [that] found that 3 percent of doctors accounted for 62 percent of opioid prescriptions."*

Pharmaceutical Companies Share the Blame for Damage Caused by the Opioid Crisis

Francie Diep

In many ways, pharmaceutical companies hold a large share of responsibility for the opioid crisis. They developed and aggressively marketed the opioid painkillers that millions of people would become addicted to. However, data suggests that most patients who used opioids for chronic pain did not develop addictions. The people who were primarily harmed by these drugs were those who misused them and often obtained them illegally. A small percentage of doctors were to blame for most illegitimate prescriptions, and they were allowed to flourish in states with little regulation. At this point in the opioid crisis, heroin and fentanyl are responsible for far more overdose deaths than prescription opioids. Francie Diep is a senior reporter at the Chronical of Higher Education.

As you read, consider the following questions:

1. According to the 2011 study of California doctors referenced in this viewpoint, what percent of doctors accounted for 62 percent of opioid prescriptions?
2. According to this viewpoint, approximately what percent of people who use opioids for chronic pain become addicted?
3. What is one potential problem that could be caused by making it more difficult to obtain prescription opioids?

P urdue Pharma, the company that makes OxyContin, has been taking some legal hits lately. Last week, the company settled a lawsuit with the state of Oklahoma for $270 million, the largest amount yet in a state opioid suit. Over the past several weeks, an ongoing case with the states of Massachusetts and New York has revealed the extent to which the Sacklers, the wealthy family that owns Purdue, were personally involved in plans to market and profit from OxyContin. Suits like these allege that Purdue advertised OxyContin as less addictive than it really is, leading to an epidemic of opioid use disorder and overdoses. Purdue and the Sacklers deny these claims.

So what's the evidence that Purdue Pharma and its marketing of OxyContin led to high rates of opioid addiction in the United States? While it's up to the courts to decide to what extent Purdue is legally responsible for America's opioid crisis, the science has been building for several years now to support the idea that the ready availability of legally manufactured, prescribed opioid painkillers was a critical force in creating the epidemic in painkiller and heroin addiction today. Below are some of the most important studies showing that link, as well as studies that illustrate the current state of the opioid epidemic.

For a Decade, as Opioid Prescriptions Rose, so Did Opioid Addiction and Deaths

In 2011, the Centers for Disease Control and Prevention (CDC) documented that, between 1999 and the late 2000s, sales of opioid painkillers—like OxyContin, Vicodin, and Percocet—quadrupled. At the same time, overdose deaths involving opioids almost quadrupled, and the proportion of people showing up in addiction treatment centers saying they had an opioid addiction went up 600 percent.

States helped provide a natural experiment showing the effect of painkiller sales on misuse and death. States with higher-than-average opioid sales tended to have higher-than-average death rates, too, the CDC found. Unscrupulous "pill mill" doctors could have a big effect on the painkiller supply in some states, CDC researchers argued, pointing to a 2011 study of California doctors who treat injured workers. That study found that 3 percent of doctors accounted for 62 percent of opioid prescriptions.

More Aggressive Opioid Marketing Is Associated with More Opioid Prescribing and Overdoses

Long after the CDC published its first figures showing how overdose deaths rose along with opioid prescriptions, a new study, published earlier this year, found that, the more money pharmaceutical companies spent on marketing opioids to doctors in a county, the more opioids doctors in that county would prescribe. Opioid overdose deaths were associated with marketing spending as well.

A Minority of People Who Are Prescribed Opioid Painkillers for Chronic Pain Become Addicted

In a review, Nora Volkow, the head of the National Institute on Drug Abuse, and Thomas McLellan, a former deputy director of the Office of National Drug Control Policy, estimated that about 8 percent of people who take prescribed opioids for chronic pain become addicted. About 15 to 26 percent act in ways that doctors consider unhealthy, but may not qualify as addiction, such as aggressively hounding doctors for prescriptions and taking more pills than they're supposed to.

Others Began Their Opioid Misuse and Addictions by Taking Prescribed Pills that Weren't Intended for Them

People with addictions to opioid painkillers are often lumped together with people with addictions to heroin because the chemicals are similar, produce similar feelings, and misuse of one can lead to misuse of the other (more on that below). But the large majority of Americans who misuse opioids take pills only, according to the latest figures from the National Survey on Drug Use and Health.

The most common source of pills for misusers is "from a relative or friend for free," according to an analysis by the Substance Abuse and Mental Health Services Administration. Together with the CDC data about high opioid prescribing rates in America, this study suggests generous prescriptions led to a ready supply of pills that people gave to their friends and family, who then used them for non-medical reasons (although the majority of respondents to the 2016 National Survey on Drug Use and Health said they misused pills to deal with pain).

A Crackdown on Pills Can Lead to Heroin Use

Because heroin is chemically similar to opioid painkillers, and will relieve withdrawal symptoms, people who are cut off from their pill supply for some reason may turn to heroin instead. One of the earlier pieces of research to demonstrate this was published in 2012, when researchers interviewed 103 people with opioid addictions. At the time, Purdue had recently introduced a version of OxyContin that was difficult to crush and dissolve in water for injection. Interviewees said they definitely preferred the old Oxy, and two-thirds said they disliked the new Oxy so much, they'd moved on to another opioid, most commonly heroin. "Most people that I know don't use OxyContin to get high anymore," one interviewee said. "They have moved on to heroin [because] it is easier to use, much cheaper, and easily available."

Journalist Sam Quinones' book *Dreamland* also documented this phenomenon.

Pharmacy Chains Held Responsible for Their Role in the Opioid Crisis

Three US pharmacy chains have recklessly distributed massive amounts of painkiller pills in two counties in Ohio.

A federal jury made this ruling on Tuesday in a verdict that could set the tone for the US city and county governments that want to hold pharmacies accountable for their roles in the opioid epidemic.

The Lake and Trumbull counties blamed CVS, Walgreens, and Walmart pharmacies for not stopping the flood of pills that caused hundreds of overdose deaths and cost each of the two counties about $1 billion (€893 million), their attorney said.

"The law requires pharmacies to be diligent in dealing drugs. This case should be a wake-up call that failure will not be accepted," said Mark Lanier, an attorney for the counties.

"The jury sounded a bell that should be heard through all pharmacies in America," Lanier added.

Attorneys for the three pharmacy chains maintained they had policies to stem the flow of pills when their pharmacists had any concerns and would notify authorities about suspicious orders from doctors.

They also said it was the doctors who controlled how many pills were being prescribed for legitimate medical needs.

It was the first time pharmacy companies had completed a trial to defend themselves in a drug crisis that has killed at least one-half-million Americans in the last twenty years.

How much the pharmacies must pay in damages will be decided by a federal judge next year.

"US Jury Holds Three Pharmacies Responsible for Opioid Crisis Killing 500,000," Euronews, November 24, 2021.

Prescriptions Have Been Falling Lately, but Overdoses Are Still Rising

After nearly a decade of studies demonstrating opioid painkillers' risks, America's doctors seem to be slowing their prescribing. In 2017, the CDC reported that the number of scripts doctors wrote for opioids fell 13 percent between 2012 and 2015, although they remain much higher than in 1999.

Yet opioid-related overdose deaths continue to rise, reaching nearly 48,000 in 2017.

Now the Deadliest Opioids Are Likely Street Drugs, Not Prescribed Pills

The most common cause of fatal opioid overdoses is now fentanyl, a very strong opioid that is available by prescription. However, officials believe much of what's killing people comes not from pharmaceutical companies, but from illicit labs in China and Mexico. Drug traffickers may mix illicitly produced fentanyl with other drugs, such as cocaine, or press it into counterfeit pills.

> *"Yet as deplorably as Sackler family members are alleged to have behaved, this epidemic was too complex for one group to have created. None of this would have been possible without us—American healthcare consumers."*

Accountability for the Opioid Crisis Is Complicated Because Many Are Culpable

Sam Quinones

According to Sam Quinones, in the early- to mid-2010s it was rare for people to openly speak about opioid addiction, despite how many lives were touched by it. It was also rare for people to file lawsuits against opioid manufacturers like Purdue Pharma. But as time passed people stopped being silent about the devastating effects of opioid use. Individuals and state attorneys general started to file lawsuits against Purdue Pharma and the Sacklers, which led to the company being forced to pay billions of dollars for the damage they have done. However, Quinones argues that despite its major role, Purdue Pharma is not solely to blame. The American healthcare system and its consumers also helped create this crisis. Sam Quinones is an independent journalist and author of four books of narrative nonfiction.

Op-Ed: Who is responsible for the opioid crisis, and who ultimately pays?" by Sam Quinones, appeared in LA Times, July 18, 2021. Reprinted by permission of the author.

As you read, consider the following questions:

1. Where is the Bottoms neighborhood, referenced in this viewpoint, located?
2. How many state attorneys general filed lawsuits against Purdue Pharma and the Sacklers?
3. Approximately how much money did the Sacklers take from Purdue Pharma overall, according to Sam Quinones?

In 2013, I was researching a book about the opioid epidemic and found myself with a lawyer touring a neighborhood known as the Bottoms in the town of Lucasville in southern Ohio.

The Bottoms is a neighborhood of poor people living in trailers and small, rough houses, and it is flooded every so often by the Scioto River, which runs nearby. Among the things that had mangled the lives of folks in the Bottoms was addiction to what everyone by then called "OC." OC was an abbreviation for OxyContin, the narcotic prescription pain pill sold with what we now know was historic flagrancy by the Connecticut company Purdue Pharma, owned by the Sackler family.

From the Bottoms had come some of the country's first plaintiffs in lawsuits against Purdue. However, none of these nor other lawsuits had prospered; opioids had a way of turning every plaintiff into what a jury would view as a conniving, thieving, child-neglecting junkie.

Meanwhile, few families anywhere, of any economic class, wanted to speak about their loved ones' addictions, their repeated treatments, their street lives and overdose deaths. They were ashamed and they hid, certain that they were alone.

So I remember walking the Bottoms convinced that the Sacklers were impervious to legal reproach. They were anonymous members of the American One Percent. Forbes later named them one of the country's wealthiest families, eclipsing the Rockefellers, due entirely, the magazine reported, to sales of the OC that damaged folks in the Bottoms of Lucasville, Ohio.

Indeed, by the time my book—"Dreamland: The True Tale of America's Opiate Epidemic"—was released in April 2015, I was used to national silence on the issue. I knew of only three lawsuits against the drug companies that sold opioids—brought by counties and on hold.

Then, to my astonishment, the silence broke. That year, families began to emerge from the shadows. Obituaries began to tell the truth. Soon lawsuits against drug companies ballooned to more than 2,600, including one from every attorney general in the country. Massachusetts was the first to sue the Sacklers by name, and other states followed.

I remembered the Bottoms when I heard the recent resolution to lawsuits brought by 15 state attorneys general. Purdue, as we know it, would cease to exist. The family would put up $4.5 billion to those states for treatment and prevention. Many millions of internal documents from Purdue and its Sackler-dominated board would be made public online.

Massachusetts Atty. Gen. Maura Healey had led this group of states. She blamed the "billionaire Sacklers" for creating the opioid epidemic through aggressive sales of OC, calling them "villains for the history books."

OxyContin helped ignite the new heroin market that expanded as prescription pain pills spread coast to coast. Before OC, opioids came mixed with acetaminophen to lessen the chance of abuse. Acetaminophen did damage to the liver and kidneys, so most folks never developed an addiction desperate enough to send them to heroin. Until OxyContin. It came with no abuse deterrent and took patients up to high daily doses very quickly. Once they lost their insurance or a doctor cut them off, they had nowhere to turn but to cheap, potent Mexican heroin.

The Sacklers, meanwhile, took hundreds of millions of dollars from Purdue every year—some $4 billion in total—which the company could have used to fund R&D and diversify away from opioids. Yet no amount of cash seemed ever enough for the Sackler board members. They flogged their sales force to ever-greater effort.

Key to all this, as well, I believe, is a healthcare system that incentivizes profitable pills and pill-taking over wellness. Purdue was hardly alone; many other companies are culpable as well. Still, it was Purdue and the Sacklers who took a product—an opioid—that is capable of miraculous good and hawked it like an over-the-counter medication.

Across America, people with enough to deal with watched as loved ones grew addicted and died from drugs intended as treatment for work injuries, car accidents, or wisdom tooth extractions.

My hunch is that the millions more documents to be made public will further pixelate that story.

To me, the Sacklers personified the Opioid Era in America—our latest Gilded Age, in which the pursuit of money was divorced from any moral compass or concern for town and neighborhood.

Yet as deplorably as Sackler family members are alleged to have behaved, this epidemic was too complex for one group to have created. None of this would have been possible without us—American healthcare consumers. Part of the story, say doctors I've spoken to, was that we pushed back when they suggested we didn't need narcotics for a lot of what ailed us, that we needed to work at our own wellness. We didn't want to hear it. We too were part of the Opioid Era.

In a larger sense, the epidemic's deeper roots lie in our isolation and our destruction of community—in wealthy neighborhoods and poor ones alike. We spent 40 years shredding community, exalting the private sector. We watched as jobs left and towns staggered, defenseless to whatever came next, which turned out, by the late 1990s, to be pain pills prescribed by doctors. All of us were made as vulnerable as those workers and the communities from which the opioid epidemic spread.

The money Purdue Pharma and the Sackler family are putting up seems to me small potatoes given the incalculable damage. Opioid addiction, meanwhile, has morphed into an epidemic of addiction to synthetic drugs produced in Mexico.

Still, despite its limitations, the Purdue Pharma settlement is an example of legal change created by grass-roots pressure, in part from typically voiceless places like southern Ohio.

Within it is the epidemic's most important lesson: Our defense against economic forces like Purdue Pharma is to understand that we are best together—out of the shadows and in community.

For it's a radical thing: what happens when people stand up to power and step into the open, understanding that they are not alone.

> "The settlement has incensed opioid activists and many legal scholars, who describe the outcome as a miscarriage of justice."

The Sackler Family Keeps Trying to Buy Their Way out of Legal Accountability for the Opioid Crisis

Brian Mann

At the time this viewpoint was published in 2017, a judge had approved a bankruptcy settlement for Purdue Pharma that would involve the Sackler family paying billions of dollars and forfeiting their ownership of Purdue Pharma in exchange for being freed from legal liability for the opioid crisis. Though Purdue Pharma as a company could be held liable, under this deal the family that owned it would not be legally responsible. Since that time, there has been much back-and-forth over the terms of the Purdue Pharma bankruptcy settlement, including the amount of money the Sacklers would pay and what legal liability they could face. However, many are outraged that these deals always involve legal immunity for the Sacklers. Brian Mann is a journalist with NPR.

As you read, consider the following questions:

1. What are the terms of the 2017 bankruptcy settlement mentioned in this viewpoint?
2. Approximately how much money had the Sacklers made from opioid sales at the time this viewpoint was published?
3. At the time this viewpoint was published, how many times had the Sacklers been charged with criminal wrongdoing?

Members of the Sackler family who are at the center of the nation's deadly opioid crisis have won sweeping immunity from opioid lawsuits linked to their privately owned company Purdue Pharma and its OxyContin medication.

Federal Judge Robert Drain approved a bankruptcy settlement on Wednesday that grants the Sacklers "global peace" from any liability for the opioid epidemic.

"This is a bitter result," Drain said. "I believe that at least some of the Sackler parties have liability for those [opioid OxyContin] claims. ... I would have expected a higher settlement."

The complex bankruptcy plan, confirmed by Drain at a hearing in White Plains, N.Y., was negotiated in a series of intense closed-door mediation sessions over the past two years.

The deal grants "releases" from liability for harm caused by OxyContin and other opioids to the Sacklers, hundreds of their associates, as well as their remaining empire of companies and trusts.

In return, they have agreed to pay roughly $4.3 billion, while also forfeiting ownership of Purdue Pharma.

In his bench ruling, Drain acknowledged the devastating harm caused by Purdue Pharma's opioid products, which he said contributed to a "massive public health crisis."

According to Drain, this settlement offers an opportunity to help communities with funding for drug treatment and other opioid abatement programs.

"It is clear to me after a lengthy trial that there is now no other reasonably conceivable means to achieve this result," he said.

The Sacklers, who admit no wrongdoing and who by their own reckoning earned more than $10 billion from opioid sales, will remain one of the wealthiest families in the world.

Representatives of the Mortimer Sackler branch of the family sent a statement to NPR.

"While we dispute the allegations that have been made about our family, we have embraced this path in order to help combat a serious and complex public health crisis."

In his ruling, Judge Drain noted that members of the Sackler family had declined to offer an explicit apology for their role leading Purdue Pharma.

"A forced apology is not really an apology," Drain said. "So we will have to live without one."

Critics of this bankruptcy settlement, meanwhile, said they would challenge Drain's confirmation because of the liability releases for the Sacklers.

"This order is insulting to victims of the opioid epidemic who had no voice in these proceedings—and must be appealed," said Washington state Attorney General Bob Ferguson on Twitter.

The U.S. Trustee Program, a division of the Justice Department that serves as a bankruptcy watchdog, also announced that it would seek a stay of Judge Drain's ruling pending the resolution of appeals.

Activists Are Outraged

The settlement has incensed opioid activists and many legal scholars, who describe the outcome as a miscarriage of justice.

"I've never seen any such abuse of justice," said Nan Goldin, an artist who emerged as a leading opioid activist after becoming addicted to OxyContin.

Goldin spoke to NPR ahead of the ruling, when it became clear Drain would approve liability releases for the Sacklers.

"It's shocking. It's really shocking. I've been deeply depressed and horrified," she said.

In a series of legal briefs and during a bankruptcy trial over the last two weeks, the Department of Justice urged Drain to reject the settlement. Attorneys general for nine states and the District of Columbia also opposed the plan.

They argued the settlement would unfairly deny individuals and governments the right to sue the Sacklers, who themselves never filed for bankruptcy protection.

"Due process requires that those with litigation claims have reasonable opportunity to be heard," argued DOJ attorney Paul Schwartzberg during the trial.

Attorneys for Purdue Pharma and the Sacklers argued that without this deal there would be legal chaos as thousands of individuals lawsuits move forward against the company and members of the family.

During the trial, Judge Drain seemed to endorse that legal argument.

In his ruling, Drain did narrow the scope of legal protections available for the Sacklers and their associates.

Consultants and advisers who worked with Purdue Pharma, including a law firm operated by former Alabama Sen. Luther Strange, will no longer be covered by the liability releases.

Attorneys for the family also demanded that family members receive protection from all lawsuits relating to their private company. Drain, however, demanded that most non-opioid claims be excluded from the deal.

He also clarified on Wednesday that protection from civil lawsuits granted to members of the Sackler family does not protect them from any criminal charges.

The Sacklers Have Never Been Charged and Say They Did Nothing Wrong

Critics say the introduction of OxyContin in the late 1990s when members of the Sackler family served on the company's board helped usher in the opioid crisis.

More than 500,000 people in the United States have died from drug overdoses involving opioids, and millions more suffer from opioid use disorder.

Purdue Pharma has pleaded guilty twice to criminal wrongdoing in its marketing of OxyContin, first in 2007 and again last year. The Sacklers have never been charged and say they did nothing illegal or unethical.

Facing a wave of negative publicity linked to their company, however, the Sacklers have seen their name stripped from buildings and institutions. Many philanthropic and cultural groups around the world have stopped accepting donations from the family.

Supporters of the bankruptcy plan—including most state and local government officials across the U.S.—have voiced unhappiness with liability releases granted to the Sacklers.

But they say the deal is expected to distribute more than $5 billion over the next decade to public trusts created to fund drug treatment and health care programs.

"Instead of years of value-destructive litigation, including between and among creditors, this plan ensures that billions of dollars will be devoted to helping people and communities who have been hurt by the opioid crisis," said Steve Miller, who chairs Purdue Pharma's board of directors, in a statement sent to NPR.

Even some early critics of the bankruptcy plan, including New York Attorney General Letitia James, said the money contributed by the Sacklers will do real good.

"No deal is perfect, and no amount of money will ever make up for the hundreds of thousands who lost their lives, the millions who became addicted, or the countless families torn apart by this crisis, but these funds will be used to prevent future death and destruction as a result of the opioid epidemic," James said in a statement.

The new company that emerges from the ashes of Purdue Pharma will be allowed to continue making and selling opioid products, including OxyContin.

But architects of this deal say future opioid profits will go to help fund drug treatment programs.

Purdue Pharma itself will re-emerge from bankruptcy as a new company operated as a form of public trust corporation.

An Appeal by the DOJ Could Be the Final Hurdle

NPR reported on Tuesday that Purdue Pharma and its attorneys launched a behind-the-scenes pressure campaign aimed at convincing the DOJ not to challenge the plan in court.

NPR acquired an early draft of a letter distributed by the drug company to groups supportive of the bankruptcy deal.

The letter is framed as a direct appeal to DOJ officials and purports to be written by those injured by the company and members of the Sackler family.

"We collectively speak for the overwhelming majority of the state and local governments, organizations, and individuals harmed by Purdue and the Sacklers," the letter states.

There is no mention in the document of the company's role launching the effort or crafting the message.

Ryan Hampton, an opioid activist who served on a key committee negotiating the bankruptcy deal, expressed outrage at Purdue Pharma's effort.

"This letter was highly inappropriate. It was wrong," Hampton told NPR. "It was written, proposed and pushed at the eleventh hour at the beckoning of Purdue Pharma."

A DOJ spokesperson declined to comment on the drug company's efforts to influence its decision-making and would not disclose the timeline for deciding whether it will file an appeal.

Periodical and Internet Sources Bibliography

The following articles have been selected to supplement the diverse views presented in this chapter.

Leo Beletsky and Jeremiah Goulka, "Opinion: The Federal Agency That Fuels the Opioid Crisis," *New York Times*, September 17, 2018. https://www.nytimes.com/2018/09/17/opinion/drugs-dea-defund-heroin.html.

CBS News Editorial Staff, "The Opioid Epidemic: Who Is to Blame?" CBS News, June 21, 2020. https://www.cbsnews.com/news/the-opioid-epidemic-who-is-to-blame-60-minutes-2020-06-21/.

Mary Harris, "The Sacklers Get to Walk Away," *Slate*, March 21, 2022. https://slate.com/news-and-politics/2022/03/sacklers-oxycontin-opioid-crisis-purdue-pharma-bankruptcy-settlement.html.

Jan Hoffman, "Sacklers Raise Their Offer to Settle Opioid Lawsuits by More Than $1 Billion," *New York Times*, February 18, 2022. https://www.nytimes.com/2022/02/18/health/sacklers-opioids-lawsuit.html.

Dietrich Knauth and Tom Hals, "Purdue Pharma Judge Overrules DOJ to Approve $6 Bln Opioid Settlement," *Reuters*, March 9, 2022. https://www.reuters.com/legal/transactional/purdue-seeks-approval-6-billion-opioid-settlement-over-state-doj-objections-2022-03-09/.

Brian Mann, "For the First Time, Victims of the Opioid Crisis Formally Confront the Sackler Family," NPR, March 10, 2022. https://www.npr.org/2022/03/10/1085174528/sackler-opioid-victims.

Brian Mann, "US Pharmacies Are Under Trial for Their Involvement in the Opioid Crisis," NPR, October 5, 2021. https://www.npr.org/2021/10/05/1043278960/u-s-pharmacies-are-under-trial-for-their-involvement-in-the-opioid-crisis.

Mukul Mehra, "Why Opioid Addiction Will Persist Until Physicians Have a Panoramic View of Opioid Exposure," *HealthAffairs*, October 4, 2018. https://www.healthaffairs.org/do/10.1377/forefront.20180928.934819/full/.

Michael Nedelman, "Doctors Increasingly Face Charges for Patient Overdoses," *CNN Health*, July 31, 2017. https://www.cnn.com/2017/07/31/health/opioid-doctors-responsible-overdose/index.html.

Jacob James Rich, "As Purdue Pharma Takes the Fall, Don't Forget the Government's Role In the Opioid Crisis," Reason Foundation, December 22, 2020. https://reason.org/commentary/as-purdue-pharma-takes-the-fall-dont-forget-the-governments-role-in-the-opioid-crisis/.

Richard Smith, "The Opioid Crisis, the Sacklers, and the Role Played by Doctors," *BMJ Opinion*, July 21, 2021. https://blogs.bmj.com/bmj/2021/07/21/the-opioid-crisis-the-sacklers-and-the-role-played-by-doctors/.

Joanna Walters, "House of Pain: Who Are the Sacklers Under Fire in Lawsuits Over Opioids?" the *Guardian*, July 26, 2019. https://www.theguardian.com/us-news/2019/jul/26/sacklers-opioids-purdue-pharma-oxycontin-opioids.

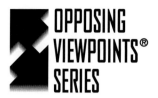

OPPOSING VIEWPOINTS® SERIES

CHAPTER 4

Can the Opioid Crisis Be Stopped?

Chapter Preface

The U.S. government and healthcare professionals have both attempted to significantly reduce the use of prescription opioids in the hope of reining in the opioid crisis. Opioid prescriptions in the U.S. have decreased by at least 40 percent in the past 10 years, with doctors increasingly turning to other methods of pain management to address postoperative and chronic pain.[1] In 2016 the US Centers for Disease Control and Prevention (CDC) issued guidelines on opioid prescribing that suggested capping the amount and duration of opioid prescriptions by doctors. In February 2022 the proposed new guidelines, which would offer more flexibility for doctors while still encouraging them to try non-opioid pain treatment options first, with opioids as a last resort in most situations.[2] But despite the steadily decreasing number of opioids being prescribed, the number of opioid overdose deaths is increasing just as steadily. According to the National Institute on Drug Abuse, the number of opioid overdose deaths rose from 21,088 in 2010 to 68,630 in 2020.[3] The COVID-19 pandemic that began in early 2020 has only made the crisis worse.

If fewer people are being prescribed opioids, then what is driving this significant increase in opioid overdose deaths? Statistics suggest the answer is fentanyl. In 2021 alone, U.S. law enforcement agencies seized 10 million fentanyl pills.[4] Since fentanyl is 30 to 50 times more potent than heroin, the risk of overdosing from intentional or unintentional ingestion is significantly higher.[5] This does not mean that finding ways to control prescription opioid abuse and addiction is pointless, since research suggests that 80 percent of people who try illegal opioids like heroin, which is commonly cut with fentanyl, start out abusing prescription opioids.[5] However, it does indicate that there is a new dimension to the opioid crisis that experts must also find a way of bringing under control.

Experts propose a variety of solutions to help bring the overdose rate down. In addition to changing the way that pain is treated and managed by healthcare professionals, some experts argue that a more nuanced approach must be taken when deciding when to prescribe opioids. Some assert that there are situations—such as when a patient has already developed an opioid dependency—where cutting off access to prescription opioids all at once may do the patient more harm than good.

According to experts in healthcare and policymaking, the laws and regulations surrounding illegal opioid possession and use may also need to be reevaluated. In 1971, the U.S. federal government began what was known as the War on Drugs, which was intended to combat illegal drug trade and use with severe penalties for people who used and distributed drugs, including incarceration.[6] Today, some are concerned that the harsh punishments for drug possession and use are helping to drive the opioid crisis. They argue that it forces the drug trade underground, where it is impossible to regulate, and deters people from seeking treatment for drug addiction. Black Americans in particular have been disproportionately harmed by the stigmatizing nature of the War on Drugs, since they have historically faced harsher punishments and higher rates of incarceration for drug-related offenses.[7]

As a result, some experts have proposed shifting away from punitive policies to those that focus on harm reduction or finding other ways to help people with substance abuse issues in a way that doesn't punish or stigmatize them. In fact, in 2021 the state of Oregon became the first to decriminalize possession of small amounts of drugs like fentanyl and heroin.[8] They are trying to shift opioid users into treatment programs rather than prison. Whether this approach is effective and will be adopted by other states remains to be seen, however. The viewpoints in this chapter consider the challenges and potential solutions to the opioid crisis from a range of perspectives.

Notes

1. Will Stone, "Pain Patients and Doctors Worry the CDC's New Opioid Guidelines May Be Damaging," NPR, April 4, 2022. https://www.npr.org/2022/04/04/1090919988/pain-patients-and-doctors-worry-the-cdcs-new-opioid-guidelines-may-be-damaging.

2.. Jan Hoffman, "CDC Proposes New Guidelines for Treating Pain, Including Opioid Use," *New York Times*, February 10, 2022. https://www.nytimes.com/2022/02/10/health/cdc-opioid-pain-guidelines.html.

3. "Overdose Death Rates," National Institute on Drug Abuse, January 20, 2022. https://nida.nih.gov/drug-topics/trends-statistics/overdose-death-rates.

4. Martin Kaste, "Fentanyl's Lethal Toll Continues. Nearly 10 Million Pills Were Seized Last Year," NPR, March 31, 2022. https://www.npr.org/2022/03/31/1089844469/fentanyls-lethal-toll-continues-police-seized-nearly-10-million-pills-last-year.

5. Michael Kim, "An opioid success story: Efforts to minimize painkillers after surgery appear to be working," the *Conversation*, September 4, 2019. https://theconversation.com/an-opioid-success-story-efforts-to-minimize-painkillers-after-surgery-appear-to-be-working-119148.

6. The Editors of Encyclopaedia Britannica "War on Drugs," *Encyclopaedia Britannica*. https://www.britannica.com/topic/war-on-drugs.

7. *Ibid.*

8. Sophie Quinton, "Oregon's Drug Decriminalization May Spread, Despite Unclear Results," the Pew Charitable Trusts, November 3, 2021. https://www.pewtrusts.org/en/research-and-analysis/blogs/stateline/2021/11/03/oregons-drug-decriminalization-may-spread-despite-unclear-results.

> *"For many people who abuse opioids, the problem begins with opioid prescriptions from their doctors for pain relief."*

Managing Pain While Reducing Opioid Use Can Help Stop the Opioid Crisis

Michael Kim

Although in recent years the majority of overdoses caused by the opioid crisis have been due to heroin and fentanyl, research shows that many people who go on to use these drugs start out misusing prescription opioids. Doctors realize they must limit the amount of opioids they prescribe to prevent more people from becoming hooked on opioids, but at the same time it is essential that they still find ways to effectively manage pain. In this viewpoint, Michael Kim examines some of the ways in which hospitals have helped reduce opioid use while addressing the issue of pain management. Michael Kim is a clinical assistant professor of anesthesiology at the Keck School of Medicine of the University of Southern California.

"An Opioid Success Story: Efforts to Minimize Painkillers After Surgery Appear to Be Working," Michael Kim, The Conversation, September 4, 2019, https://theconversation.com/an-opioid-success-story-efforts-to-minimize-painkillers-after-surgery-appear-to-be-working-119148. Licensed under CC BY-ND 4.0

As you read, consider the following questions:

1. According to this viewpoint, how did the number of deaths from opioid overdoses compare to the number of deaths from traffic accidents in 2017?
2. What percent of people who used heroin for the first time between 2016 and 2017 started with prescription drugs, according to the U.S. Department of Health and Human Services?
3. According to Michael Kim, what are some of the ways doctors can help reduce pain after surgery aside from opioid prescriptions?

The opioid epidemic has been wreaking misery and death across the nation for years. In 2017 alone, opioid overdoses killed more than 47,000 people—10,000 more deaths than were caused by traffic accidents that year.

For many people who abuse opioids, the problem begins with opioid prescriptions from their doctors for pain relief. Government data show that 21%-29% of patients who are prescribed opioids go on to misuse them, and 8% to 12% develop an opioid abuse disorder. From 2016-2017, 800,000 people used heroin for the first time, according to the U.S. Department of Health and Human Services, with 80% starting with prescription drugs.

Many hospitals have begun to take steps to minimize the amount of opioids prescribed after surgery by managing pain through alternative methods. Research suggests that these programs can reduce the need for opioids after surgery and can reduce both post-surgical complications and the average length of hospital stay.

At Keck Medicine at the University of Southern California, I'm the director of our program to reduce opioid prescriptions and manage pain in other ways. I have spent the past year leading our enhanced recovery team to design and implement various pathways that have significantly reduced the opioid burden in our surgical patients. Here's how these programs look in practice.

New Practices, Less Pain

We have modeled our program to manage pain after others that were developed originally to improve outcomes and shorten hospital stays after colorectal surgery. These programs, called Enhanced Recovery After Surgery, or ERAS, involve a range of measures, such as employing many different ways to reduce pain, and early mobility.

We have found that these protocols are easy to enact and can be as simple as giving the patients non-narcotic pain relievers in the days leading up to surgery to prep the body prior to surgery.

Some of the other methods include:

- Ensuring the patients and their families have clear understanding and expectations about post-surgical pain management
- Making sure a patient has plenty of fluids and carbohydrates
- Using a nerve block during surgery
- Encouraging the patient to get up and walking within a day after surgery
- Sending the patients home with no opioid prescriptions, or with a prescription for a very small number of pills.

We have partnered with clinicians across the health care continuum. The process involves physicians, nurses, physical therapists, occupational therapists, case management, nutrition, pre-op management and social work.

While we have not yet published the results of our programs in an academic journal, I can say that these practices produced very tangible results; the post-operative opioid usage decreased by 50% in our division of thoracic surgery and by 60% in our department of urology.

The hospital's division of cardiac surgery also reduced the use of post-operative opioid use by 45% for patients undergoing minimally invasive valve-replacement procedures. We anticipate publishing data on this finding as well. Some of our patients have gone through pre-op, surgery and post-operative care without the use of opioids at all and without any undue pain.

Other hospitals have reported success, too.

The University of Pittsburgh Medical Center cut the number of post-surgical opioid prescriptions in half.

A Cleveland Clinic pilot program to reduce opioid prescriptions in new mothers following Cesarean sections immediately reduced opioid use by two-thirds, and opioid-free hospital stays more than tripled.

A year after the University of Virginia implemented its ERAS protocol for patients undergoing thoracic surgery, it reduced the use of post-surgical morphine equivalents by more than half, reduced length of stay by two days, and even cut hospital operating costs.

These practices go beyond minimizing opioid prescriptions and can contribute to better overall patient care. For example, at Keck Medicine, our preliminary results show that we have been able to decrease the length of patient stay by up to 21% and have reduced complications from atrial fibrillation, or irregular heart beats that can lead to stroke, blood clots and heart failure, in thoracic surgery to less than 10%. We have also decreased intensive care stay for head and neck surgery by as much as one day. Also, we have cut by two days the length of time that catheters need to remain inserted into the bladders of post-operative urological patients. This is important because the risk of infection increases the longer a catheter remains inserted.

Advocating for Patients

Consulting with patients before surgery can help them understand how to deal with post-surgical pain in different ways.

An integral piece of the success is patient education. Most patients are so overwhelmed when they are about to undergo surgery and may be unaware that there are procedures to help limit opioid usage. And those who hear about opioid-minimizing practices may fear potential post-operative pain and may not consider that option.

It is important to educate patients well before their surgeries so they know their expected level of pain after their surgery and the different medication and procedures in place to minimize that post-operative pain. This kind of education is key in empowering patients to make informed decisions regarding opioids and their health.

> "The international data thus suggest
> that it's not just the volume of opioid
> prescribing that matters, but where
> and how opioids are prescribed
> and used."

The U.S. Is Not the Only Country with Opioid Issues, but It Can Learn from Other Countries

Keith Humphreys, Jonathan P. Caulkins, and Vanda Felbab-Brown

This viewpoint explains the ways in which American pharmaceutical companies are fueling the opioid epidemic in other countries by lobbying for more opioid prescriptions and increased availability in these countries. However, even though some other countries are experiencing higher rates of opioid use and addiction, there are a number of lessons the U.S. can learn from abroad about managing the opioid crisis. Keith Humphreys is a professor of psychiatry and behavioral science at Stanford University. Jonathan P. Caulkins is a professor of operations research and public policy at Carnegie Mellon University. Vanda Felbab-Brown is a senior fellow in the Center for Security, Strategy, and Technology at the Brookings Institute.

"What the US and Canada Can Learn from Other Countries to Combat the Opioid Crisis," by Keith Humphreys, Jonathan P. Caulkins, and Vanda Felbab-Brown, The Brookings Institution, January 13, 2020. Reprinted by permission.

As you read, consider the following questions:

1. What are some of the other countries that are experiencing an increase in opioid prescribing?
2. How does the number of opioid prescriptions in France compare to the U.S., according to this viewpoint?
3. What are the five lessons listed in this viewpoint that the U.S. can learn from other countries?

In a 2018 article for Foreign Affairs, we detailed what set off the North American opioid crisis and what other nations can learn from mistakes the U.S. and Canada made. Here, we describe the opioid situation in other countries and then reflect on what U.S. and Canadian officials could learn from them. Key lessons include that flooding the health care system with prescription opioids isn't necessary to manage the population's pain, guaranteed health care access may help slow opioid epidemics, and the rules for how opioids are prescribed matter, among others.

Unscrupulous U.S. Pharma Companies Are Exporting the Opioid Epidemic Abroad

Opioid prescribing in multiple Western countries (e.g. the Netherlands, the United Kingdom, Israel) has risen significantly over the past decade, though not yet to U.S. levels. The more explosive growth is in middle- and low-income countries.

Much of the new growth is fueled by U.S. companies, including Mundipharma, which like Purdue Pharma is owned by the Sackler family. Purdue drove early stages of the U.S. opioid crisis by promoting OxyContin in misleading and unethical ways, notably misrepresenting its risk of addiction when used to treat chronic, non-cancer pain. Likewise, Mundipharma has actively lobbied to open up European countries to greater opioid prescribing, as well as sponsored doctors to promote prescription opioids and deny their high potential for addiction. It has also set up and financed ostensibly patient-led groups to advocate greater access to opioids. In Poland, this has produced new legislation allowing any doctor, not merely specialty pain doctors, to write opioid prescriptions. In Italy, Mundipharma's business practices have already triggered police and legal investigations. Some Western European companies, such as Germany's Grunenthal, have copied Mundipharma's tactics.

Mundipharma has also set up joint ventures with powerful pharmaceutical companies in developing countries with huge populations, such as India and Brazil. These joint ventures have great potential to cause addiction around the globe, as they already operate supply networks in their countries and broader regions and have extensive experience in lobbying governments and populations. India's pharmaceutical industry has been weakly regulated, with an even higher capacity for policy and regulatory capture than has afflicted the United States. As an important driver of India's economic growth and job generation, the pharmaceutical industry exercises powerful influence on India's government. It has lately been pressuring the government of Narendra Modi to raise ceilings on drug prices and expand support for its activities abroad. India has substantial undertreated pain; if India's pharmaceutical companies embrace Western-supplied opioids or produce their own generic morphine primarily for acute or cancer pain, that would not be problematic. However, from Delhi to Mumbai to Kolkata, for-profit pain clinics are proliferating, and addiction is rising. Small and large Indian companies sell powerful opioids for all kinds of pain. Some employ legal tricks to avoid regulations, and some engage in frankly illegal diversion. In Brazil, already reeling from a decade-old crack cocaine epidemic, prescriptions for opioid painkillers grew by 465% in six years.

The joint ventures with Indian firms also give U.S. pharma companies access to markets across the Middle East and Africa. Pain is critically under-medicated in those regions, but corruption in the pharmacy system often results in opioids feeding addiction rather than only being used compassionately. In Nigeria, for example, tramadol in theory requires a prescription; but a less than $10 bribe in a pharmacy will enable a customer to buy it because of pervasive corruption and poor law enforcement. Similar problems are evident in other nations, including Iraq and Lebanon.

China and India Remain Obstacles to Controlling Illicit Synthetic Opioids

Meanwhile, China has historically exerted minimal control over producers of illicit fentanyl and other synthetic opioids. Under U.S. pressure, it "scheduled" all analogs of fentanyl in 2019— meaning that their production and export now are regulated and require special permits. But Beijing's capacity to enforce the new rules remains limited, and—in the midst of ongoing rancor with the United States—its motivation to do so may be lacking as well. Although at least 5,000 pharmaceutical and 160,000 chemical companies operate hundreds of thousands of production facilities, it only has some 2,000 inspectors who conduct as few as 600 inspections per year. China could tighten controls by increasing the number of inspectors, conducting sting operations and unannounced inspections, and mandating that all facilities have 100% close-circuit TV coverage monitored by independent inspectors. But boosting capacity along those lines requires will, and China may not find that will until more of its own population becomes addicted to pharmaceutically produced opioids. As of now, China's users still mostly consume heroin and methamphetamine from Myanmar, with cocaine from Latin America being the new exciting fad.

What the United States and Canada Can Learn from Other Countries

If the rest of the world is thus far not learning much from U.S. and Canadian policy failures, can the latter learn from the former? We offer five such lessons.

Lesson 1: Flooding the health care system with prescription opioids is not needed for population pain management.

Pharmaceutical companies and patient advocacy groups (some of which are industry-funded) argue that the near-quadrupling of opioid prescribing that began in the mid-1990s was a necessary response to an extraordinary level of pain in the population. But there is no evidence that the United States, which after all has one of the youngest populations in the developed world, experiences more pain than other countries. Neither is there any evidence that the explosion of opioid prescribing that began in the mid-1990s reduced population pain in the U.S.

Meanwhile France, the developed country which population pain surveys indicate is most similar to the United States, consumes barely one-fifth the prescription opioids on a per capita basis. The U.S. high prescribing level is not a necessary consequence of its level of population pain.

Lesson 2: Guaranteed health care access may, paradoxically, help slow opioid epidemics.

Limits to accessing care can make the epidemic worse. The structure of insurance benefits in the U.S. often incentivizes prescribing (relatively cheap) opioids over the more extended care an individual may need (e.g., a course of physical therapy, orthodontic surgery, extended mental health treatment). The U.S. practice of tying high-quality health insurance to employment—unique among developed countries—often means that severely addicted people will not get substance use disorder (SUD) treatment because they cannot obtain or hold down such jobs. Furthermore, the patchwork system of uncoordinated providers and payers makes it easier for people with SUD to obtain multiple prescriptions from different sources ("doctor shop"), sometimes to the point of being able to sell pills to others. Adopting one of the universal coverage approaches present in other developed nations, including universal health care records, could help the U.S. address these challenges.

Lesson 3: The rules under which opioids are prescribed matter.

The number-one per capita consumer of opioids in the world is the U.S., and Canada is third. Germany is second, but by all accounts it does not have an opioid epidemic. Why not?

Germany's high per capita opioid consumption rate is driven by extensive use of opioids in institutional settings (e.g., fentanyl during inpatient surgery). But unlike in Canada and the United States, in Germany prescriptions for chronic non-cancer pain are uncommon for people living outside of medical facilities. Only 4.5% of Germans living in the community receive an opioid prescription each year, versus 20% of Canadians. This means that in Germany, there is far less medically unsupervised opioid use and far fewer opioid pills accumulating in medicine cabinets, where they can be accessed by people other than the intended patient.

The international data thus suggest that it's not just the volume of opioid prescribing that matters, but where and how opioids are prescribed and used. It was the combination of expanded prescribing under conditions of minimal patient oversight that proved problematic in the U.S. and Canada.

Lesson 4: Fentanyl supply can sometimes remain regional, not universal.

People who become addicted to prescription opioids often "trade down" to purchase opioids from illegal markets. In parts of North America, this now presents a high risk of being exposed to extremely deadly synthetic opioids, such as fentanyl, which dealers increasingly use to adulterate heroin and counterfeit opioid pills in those regions.

So far, synthetic opioids are common in only some North American markets. As a recent RAND report observed, 9,000 more Americans would die each year if the per capita rate of synthetic opioid-related deaths in the rest of the country rose to even half what it was in New England in 2017. The geography is similar but reversed in Canada, where western not eastern provinces—notably British Columbia and Alberta—are the most severely affected.

Markets in more regions might embrace synthetic opioids, amplifying death rates, because fentanyl costs wholesale drug dealers only about 1% as much per morphine-equivalent dose as does heroin. However, the sharp east-west gaps now seen in Canada and the U.S. may persist. After all, many countries' illegal markets do not yet have fentanyl, but could. For example, when heroin markets were disrupted in 2001 and Estonia got fentanyl, its neighbor Finland got (black-market) buprenorphine instead. Finland's black-market suppliers eschewed fentanyl for no obvious reason, but fentanyl has now been entrenched in Estonia for nearly 20 years, while remaining rare just 50 miles away in Finland. Unsurprisingly, Finland's drug-related death rates remain well below those in Estonia.

A moral for the U.S. and Canada is not to give up hope that strong efforts might block fentanyl's spread and spare some regions from suffering the horrific death rates now observed in British Columbia, New England, and Appalachia.

Lesson 5: Once synthetic opioids become entrenched, they tend to persist.

Local outbreaks of synthetic opioids sometimes fizzle, but there is essentially no example of a major market where synthetic opioids disappeared after becoming entrenched. In the words of the RAND report, synthetic opioids' spread may be episodic, but it has ratchet-like persistence.

That is understandable. Synthetic opioids present a more elusive target for law enforcement than does heroin. Unlike opioids derived from poppy crops, synthetic opioids can be produced anywhere, and in small, indoor operations. Some of them are so extraordinarily potent—at least 25 times as potent, per gram, as heroin—that the quantities transported are much smaller.

This suggests that although regions that have not yet been heavily affected have good reason to try to resist incursions, once synthetic opioids have become established, efforts to root out that supply may be quixotic.

We see evidence that prescription opioid led crises are being fomented in multiple regions around the world, perhaps sending more countries down the agonizing path trod by the United States and Canada. Neither the U.S. approach to drug policy nor the very different approach in Canada has been able to prevent very large increases in opioid overdose deaths. However, we have described five lessons from abroad that the U.S., Canada, and these additional regions might apply to lessen the destruction of their ongoing epidemics.

> *"Removing access to opioids altogether isn't the solution. There are individuals suffering from chronic pain who need or strongly benefit from these drugs."*

Opioids Can Be Made Harder to Abuse

Zaina Qureshi

Pain is a major issue in the United States. Millions of people suffer from acute pain, and many are in genuine need of painkillers like opioids to help manage this pain. For this reason, to simply stop prescribing opioids would create more problems. One possible solution is to make formulation changes to opioid drugs to make them less addictive or change the way they are administered so people can only use them under medical supervision. Monitoring drug prescriptions is another way to prevent opioid abuse, and directly consulting with patients about how they would like to manage their pain could also help. Zaina Qureshi is an assistant professor of health services policy and management at the University of South Carolina.

As you read, consider the following questions:

1. What is one idea the FDA has come up with to deter opioid abuse, as mentioned in the viewpoint?
2. What do prescription drug monitoring programs do?
3. What does the author suggest measuring in addition to the amount of pain a patient feels?

How can we combat the opioid epidemic?

One of the government's most recent suggestions is to take Opana ER, an opioid indicated for very severe pain, off the market. The request, filed by the U.S. Food and Drug Administration in June, was linked to concerns of abuse-related HIV and hepatitis C outbreaks.

But removing access to opioids altogether isn't the solution. There are individuals suffering from chronic pain who need or strongly benefit from these drugs. The National Center for Health Statistics estimates that a fourth of the nation's population suffers from pain lasting longer than 24 hours. Millions more suffer from acute pain.

As a researcher who studies how pharmaceuticals are used and what effects they have, I believe it makes more sense to reduce both the supply and demand side of prescription drug abuse—without interfering with their safe and appropriate use. We can do this by reimagining how we design and prescribe addictive drugs.

Redesigning the Pill

Opioids such as morphine typically relieve pain by acting on opioid receptors distributed throughout the central nervous system.

The FDA has come up with a number of ways to deter abuse by changing the way drugs work. For example, manufacturers could include an opioid antagonist in the formulation. This is essentially a drug that blocks the opioid's effect by binding to the same receptors in the brain that the opioid would. Changing the

The U.S. Department of Health and Human Services' Plan to Fight the Opioid Crisis

HHS has a comprehensive strategy to empower local communities on the frontlines. The opioid epidemic is one of the Department's top priorities.

1. Access: Better Prevention, Treatment, and Recovery Services

HHS issued over $800 million in grants in 2017 to support treatment, prevention, and recovery, while making it easier for states to receive waivers to cover treatment through their Medicaid programs. (Issued 5 such SUD waivers since PHE declaration.)

2. Data: Better Data on the Epidemic

HHS is improving our understanding of the crisis by supporting more timely, specific public health data and reporting, including through accelerating CDC's reporting of drug overdose data.

3. Pain: Better Pain Management

HHS wants to ensure everything we do—payments, prescribing guidelines, and more — promotes healthy, evidence-based methods of pain management.

4. Overdoses: Better Targeting of Overdose-Reversing Drugs

HHS works to better target the availability of lifesaving overdose-reversing drugs. The President's 2019 Budget includes $74 million in new investments to support this goal.

5. Research: Better Research on Pain and Addiction

HHS supports cutting edge research on pain and addiction, including through a new NIH public-private partnership.

"HHS 5-Point Strategy to Combat the Opioid Crisis," National Association of Emergency Medical Technicians, August 22, 2018.

formulation in this way would reduce the chances of experiencing the euphoric high that leads to addiction.

A good example of an opioid that does this is Targiniq ER. If Targiniq ER is crushed or dissolved, it releases Naloxone, an opioid antagonist that blocks the effect of the opioid.

Another option is to redesign the drug so it must be injected or implanted, instead of taken orally. That way, the drug would potentially have to be delivered under medical supervision. Requiring the drugs to be delivered under medical supervision could also potentially reduce the improper use of needles and related outbreaks.

Even so, no method is foolproof; abusers can sometimes manipulate a changed drug. For example, Opana ER was designed to be difficult to crush, but abusers began to dissolve the drug into a solution and injecting it. To deter drug abuse, Opana ER's manufacturer, Endo Pharmaceuticals, devised a new medication formula that made the coating more difficult to crush or dissolve. Unfortunately, abusers still found a way to remove the coating and inject the drug.

Required Prescription Monitoring

Prescription drug monitoring programs have shown considerable promise in tracking potential abusers.

These programs provide emergency departments and physicians with information about a patient's past use of controlled substances at the point of care. This can immediately flag any potential for abuse, making the doctor's decision to prescribe opioids—or not— much easier.

Now, the U.S. Substance Abuse and Mental Health Services Administration has funded at least nine states to combine their prescription monitoring programs with local hospital electronic health records and other systems already in place. These collaborations provide clinicians with a comprehensive history of controlled substance, so they can make informed decisions about patient health.

This has already had some success. For example, Illinois saw a 22 percent decrease in number of opioid prescriptions issued by prescribers and a 41 percent decrease in the number of patients who received at least one opioid prescription.

More information on the nature of the epidemic—particularly its link to rural areas—could yield clues about where and how to intervene. However, publicly available data have limited geographical information and don't cover all information we might need, such as data about dose or treatment duration. What data are available are restricted to protect the identity of individuals.

Rather than look at patients with opioid issues, we decided to look at the doctors who prescribe the drugs. Our group has been working with the state of South Carolina to combine our prescription drug monitoring program, called South Carolina Reporting and Identification Prescription Tracking System, or SCRIPTS, with Medicaid data.

While we were able to combine only two years' worth of data, our research led to important insights into the abuse potential within South Carolina.

By geocoding state prescription information, we found that a relatively small percentage of providers, concentrated in a few counties, accounted for most opioid prescriptions. In 2010, the top 10 percent of prescribers wrote more than half of all opioid prescriptions.

This group represents a potential target for physician education and engagement in handling pain management and appropriate use of opioids.

Rethinking How We Assess Patients

Many solutions to the opioid crisis tend to focus on how far it has come and how to mitigate it. However, a more sustainable approach would be to rethink the process of care and engage the patient—who is at the center of it all.

When patients are engaged in the care process, they tend to adhere more to their prescribed regimens and experience better health outcomes.

In most primary care settings, it is considered standard practice to ask patients to rate their pain on a scale from one to 10. This is a very crude measure, but now we need a more sophisticated method. Medical care should consider not only the providers' preferences, but the patient's, too.

We need a tool that gets at not only the level of pain an individual experiences, but also their preferences in dealing with pain. Studies show that patient-provider communication plays an important role in pain management. If patients could share their specific concerns regarding their pain and their goals for treatment, then clinicians would be able to find the best treatment plan that is tailored to individual patient preferences.

Rather than using a standardized approach that matches pain level to doses of an analgesic or opioid, clinicians should assess each patient individually, looking at their tolerance for pain, their priorities for treatment and how they value outcomes.

By centering pain management on individual patients, we can give them a voice in the decision-making process. Given the issues with opioid abuse, I think such a pain management tool would yield a multitude of benefits, such as cutting down unnecessary prescriptions, matching the therapy to the patient's needs and improving outcomes.

"Safe injection sites are built on the premise that our goal should be to reduce the harm caused by drugs— not to punish those who use them."

Safe Injection Sites Save Lives

Trace Mitchell

In the following viewpoint Trace Mitchell argues that the opioid crisis can be mitigated by the availability of safe injection sites. However, the U.S. Department of Justice disagrees, vowing to aggressively stop the opening of such sites in the United States. Mitchell contends that the intent behind the DOJ's opposition is that drug use should be treated as a crime rather than a public health issue. Trace Mitchell is a Research Assistant with the Liberty and Law Center at George Mason University. His work has appeared in the Hill, RealClearPolicy, American Banker, Chicago Tribune, and various other publications.

As you read, consider the following questions:

1. What is a safe injection site?
2. What is the relevance of US Code Title 21, Section 865 to safe injection sites?
3. Who is Rod Rosenstein, and what was his importance at the time this viewpoint was written?

The opioid crisis is one of the most important issues facing the United States today. In 2018, the Trump administration signed a bipartisan bill aimed at fighting the opioid crisis through coordinated action and expanded access to medical treatment.

Politicians from both sides of the aisle are extremely concerned about the rising number of opioid-related deaths—and for good reason. Approximately 130 Americans die from an opioid-related overdose every day. In 2017, the number of opioid-related overdoses was six times higher than it was in 1999. The question is no longer whether we have an opioid epidemic; it is how we address it.

Safe Injection Sites

In order to try to combat this issue, people are considering opening up safe injection sites. These are places where individuals can come to test the quality of their drugs, obtain sterile injection equipment, and inject their drugs under medical supervision.

While these sites are new to the US, they have become common practice in many other countries around the world. Canada has the oldest safe injection site in North America, Insite, which has been in operation since 2003.

Insite and efforts like it have seen fairly remarkable success. Research shows that they significantly decrease overdoses without increasing the amount of drug use. Insite has not experienced one overdose in the entire 15-year period they have been in operation.

Efforts like these are just now gaining traction in the United States. Cities like San Francisco and Philadelphia have recently made efforts to establish safe injection facilities. So why haven't they started operating yet? The answer is fairly simple: there is a strong possibility that they are currently illegal.

United States Code Title 21, Section 865, makes it unlawful to

> knowingly open, lease, rent, use, or maintain any place, whether permanently or temporarily, for the purpose of manufacturing, distributing, or using any controlled substance.

This is a fairly obscure section of the Controlled Substances Act that was added at the height of the crack epidemic and is commonly known as the "Crack House" statute. It was intended to discourage people from allowing their homes to be used for drug-related purposes.

Do They Harm Society?

So why are safe injection sites so afraid that they are violating a statute that was clearly passed for an entirely different purpose? The answer lies with the Department of Justice (DOJ).

In 2018, Rod Rosenstein, the Deputy Attorney General of the United States, published an op-ed in The New York Times titled "Fight Drug Abuse, Don't Subsidize It." In this article, Mr. Rosenstein made an argument for why he thinks safe injection sites are harmful to society. However, he did not stop with advocacy. Mr. Rosenstein specifically said that "cities and counties should expect the Department of Justice to meet the opening of any injection site with swift and aggressive action." He made it clear that anyone hoping to open and operate a safe injection site would face strong opposition from the DOJ. And he was not bluffing.

On February 5, 2019, United States Attorney William M. McSwain filed a complaint with the United States District Court for the Eastern District of Pennsylvania seeking a declaratory judgment against Safehouse, a safe injection site set to open in Philadelphia, Pennsylvania, as well as against Jeanette Bowles, its executive director. The complaint asks the court to declare safe injection sites illegal under the Controlled Substances Act. The federal government is sending a clear signal: if you try to open up a safe injection site, they will prosecute you.

So why is the federal government so against the establishment of safe injection sites? If you ask Mr. Rosenstein, it's because these sites "create serious public safety risks" and "destroy the surrounding community." However, as we have seen, the evidence leans strongly against the conclusion that safe injections sites pose more public safety risks than they alleviate or that they destroy the communities that surround them. The more likely reason for this strong opposition is that safe injection sites undermine the DOJ's position that drug use should be treated as a crime rather than a public health issue.

Safe injection sites are built on the premise that our goal should be to reduce the harm caused by drugs—not to punish those who use them. This stands in stark contrast to the DOJ's position that it is not the harm caused by drugs but drug use itself that we should work to combat. If they allow safe injection sites to open and they achieve the same success they have in the past, this would serve as a huge blow to the DOJ's current position. People may begin to think that it is the harm caused by drugs—and not drug use in and of itself—that is actually the issue.

Regardless of the true intent behind these actions, it is clear that the DOJ plans to fight safe injection sites tooth and nail. This will serve as a major hindrance for people who are trying to find evidence-based, practical solutions for combating the opioid crisis. It remains to be seen how the court will rule on safe injection sites and whether or not they violate federal law, but the DOJ's aggressive actions send a definite signal to those hoping to open up one of these facilities: expect fierce opposition.

> *"People have often turned to alcohol, opioids and other drugs to help them cope with the pandemic."*

The COVID-19 Pandemic Has Made the Opioid Crisis Worse

Dennis Thompson

As Dennis Thompson explains in this viewpoint, in some ways the COVID-19 pandemic had positive impacts on opioid treatment in the United States. It made telehealth more common and accessible to patients seeking opioid treatment, and also the federal government expanded addiction treatment coverage. However, overdose deaths increased significantly since the start of the COVID-19 pandemic in early 2020. Many people turned to opioids and other substances to cope with stresses associated with the panedemic, and because of issues with the supply chain many people who used opioids ended up consuming drugs cut with fentanyl, which increased the risk of overdosing. Dennis Thompson is a reporter for HealthDay.

As you read, consider the following questions:

1. How much did opioid overdose deaths increase between 2019 and 2020?
2. According to this viewpoint, how did supply chain issues caused by COVID-19 affect people who use opioids?
3. According to Zachary Talbott, what is one positive trend healthcare providers have observed since the start of the COVID-19 pandemic?

The COVID-19 pandemic has shaken up the U.S. opioid crisis in ways bad and good, increasing the risk of use and overdose but also spurring innovative approaches to treatment.

The pandemic has definitely been linked to an increase in opioid use and overdose deaths, Tufts University's Thomas Stopka said during a *HealthDay Now* video interview.

"We've been seeing increases in opioid overdose deaths over the past 15 to 20 years, but the increase from 2019 to 2020 was upwards of a 30% increase, from about 70,000 the previous year to 93,000 in 2020," said Stopka, an associate professor of public health and community medicine at Tufts School of Medicine in Boston.

People have often turned to alcohol, opioids and other drugs to help them cope with the pandemic, he said.

"We were all stressed out about the pandemic, and about infection coming into our neighborhoods, into our homes, into our families," Stopka said. "That seemed to have an impact on substance use practices."

For opioid users, the pandemic created an added risk by disrupting supply chains for illicit drugs, he noted. It's very similar to the way COVID-19 caused shortages in food, toilet paper and other necessities.

"Folks who might have relied on a traditional pattern of supply over many years now might have had breakage in that supply, because maybe overall supply chains were also decimated by people getting sick, people taking care of their loved ones," Stopka said. "If folks couldn't rely on their typical source of illicit opioids, then they don't know exactly what they're getting."

Opioids from new sources increase a person's risk of overdose because the drugs could be cut with more powerful substances like fentanyl, a synthetic opioid that's up to 100 times more powerful than morphine.

"People don't always know what they're getting," Stopka said. "There's a pretty good chance there's going to be fentanyl in heroin, and it might be cut with other things."

But the increase in fentanyl-tainted drugs might have contributed to another COVID-era trend—more people seeking earlier treatment at programs that have developed greater flexibility in response to pandemic-era challenges, said Zachary Talbott, president of Talbott Legacy Centers, a drug treatment program in Maryville, Tenn.

"We're having people come into treatment after a year of problematic use, whereas prior I would have people with a history of 10 years, 12 years, 15 years," Talbott said in a HealthDay Now interview. "I think in some ways the increase in overdoses—we hear this from patients across the region—has scared them."

COVID-inspired social distancing requirements also have made it easier for people to get treatment for substance use disorder, Talbott and Stopka said.

For example, the pandemic spurred a dramatic increase in telehealth services in all medical fields. People struggling with substance use particularly benefited from the ability to get remote care, the experts said.

A former opioid abuser himself, Talbott recalled that he used to drive as much as four hours a day going to and from treatment.

"That goes back to my privilege," he said. "That's not achievable for the vast majority of people who don't have a car that can make such a drive, who would have to work, don't have family or other resources."

But virtual health care isn't perfect.

"We have a lot of folks in rural areas or more impoverished areas in Appalachia that just don't have the technology or data plans to do telehealth," Talbott said.

The U.S. Centers for Medicare and Medicaid have "allowed audio only during the pandemic, but you cannot engage in follow-up in the same way—that, to me, has been limiting," Talbott continued.

"We can still do a lot of good stabilizing of the brain with medication, but it's all the stuff that comes after that that really makes for a lasting recovery plan," he said. "We struggle during the pandemic to continue to the same level."

But the availability of telehealth, combined with expanded federal coverage of addiction treatment, has made it much easier for people to get the help they need, the experts said.

Medicare and Medicaid now cover all three medications approved by the U.S. Food and Drug Administration to treat opioid use disorder, Talbott said. Those are methadone, buprenorphine and naltrexone.

To help with social distancing, the federal government also started allowing treatment centers to hand out take-home doses of the medications.

Until now, people had to go to their center every day to receive their dose of methadone, Stopka and Talbott said.

The take-home doses allowed treatment centers to more quickly and efficiently handle patients on methadone, Talbott said.

"We could stagger half of those that normally would be daily in that first early period to Monday, Wednesday and Friday, and the other half to Tuesday, Thursday, Saturday, so we could cut in half on these days the number of patients," he said. "Those that were stable on their dosage, we could go ahead and do a week even."

The concern now is that when the pandemic winds down treatment centers might lose some of this government-granted flexibility, Stopka said.

"If folks are having success with the take-home doses and having success with the telemedicine visits, and now they have to revert to going back to the clinic more frequently, then there are some folks that might not have the ability to drive to the clinic, particularly in places where you might have to drive two hours each way," Stopka said.

Periodical and Internet Sources Bibliography

The following articles have been selected to supplement the diverse views presented in this chapter.

Jan Hoffman, "C.D.C. Proposes New Guidelines for Treating Pain, Including Opioid Use," *New York Times,* February 10, 2022. https://www.nytimes.com/2022/02/10/health/cdc-opioid-pain-guidelines.html.

Abby Goodnough, "Helping Drug Users Survive, Not Abstain: 'Harm Reduction' Gains Federal Support," *New York Times,* June 27, 2021. https://www.nytimes.com/2021/06/27/health/overdose-harm-reduction-covid.html.

Christen Linke Young and Abigail Durak, "How Do We Tackle the Opioid Crisis?" Brookings Institute, October 18, 2019. https://www.brookings.edu/policy2020/votervital/how-do-we-tackle-the-opioid-crisis/.

Brian Mann, "Overdose Deaths Rose During the War on Drugs, But Efforts to Reduce Them Face Backlash," NPR, June 19, 2021. https://www.npr.org/2021/06/19/1006891729/overdose-deaths-rose-during-the-war-on-drugs-but-efforts-to-reduce-them-face-bac.

James Marson, Julie Wernau, and David Luhnow, "The Once and Future Drug War," *Wall Street Journal*, January 21, 2022. https://www.wsj.com/articles/the-once-and-future-drug-war-11642780895.

Bryce Pardo and Peter Reuter, "Enforcement Strategies for Fentanyl and Other Synthetic Opioids," Brookings Institute, June 22, 2020. https://www.brookings.edu/research/enforcement-strategies-for-fentanyl-and-other-synthetic-opioids/.

Jacob James Rich and Robert Capodilupo, "Prescription Drug Monitoring Programs: Effects on Opioid Prescribing and Drug Overdose Mortality," Reason Foundation, July 29, 2021. https://reason.org/policy-study/prescription-drug-monitoring-programs-effects-on-opioid-prescribing-and-drug-overdose-mortality/.

Hannah Schoenbaum, "Native Tribes Demand Congress Provide 'All the Resources Necessary' to Combat Opioid Crisis," the *Hill*, April 5, 2022. https://thehill.com/news/house/3259909-native-tribes-demand-congress-provide-all-the-resources-necessary-to-combat-opioid-crisis/.

Abdullah Shihipar, "An Anti-Overdose Drug Is Getting Stronger. Maybe That's a Bad Thing?" the *Atlantic*, January 14, 2022. https://www.theatlantic.com/health/archive/2022/01/naloxone-stronger-form-opioid-overdose/621254/.

Nora D. Volkow, "Making Addiction Treatment More Realistic and Pragmatic: The Perfect Should Not Be the Enemy of the Good," *HealthAffairs*, January 3, 2022. https://www.healthaffairs.org/do/10.1377/forefront.20211221.691862/.

For Further Discussion

Chapter 1

1. Based on the information about opioid use and addiction in the U.S. following the Civil War provided in the first viewpoint, what are some parallels between the opioid crisis of the late nineteenth and early twentieth centuries similar to today's opioid crisis?
2. In what ways do this chapter's arguments about why the opioid crisis started overlap with one another? In what ways do they differ?
3. Does the Sackler family deserves a harsher punishment for their role in the opioid crisis? Why or why not?

Chapter 2

1. The Pew Charitable Trusts argues that people living in rural communities face greater barriers to opioid treatment than those in urban areas, while Carla R. Jackson asserts the opposite. Which argument do you find more compelling? Explain.
2. How does gender relate to opioid use and addiction?
3. What are some of the current healthcare disparities Black patients face, and how might they be addressed?

Chapter 3

1. Do you think the U.S. federal government has done enough to prevent and stop the opioid crisis? Explain your reasoning.
2. Does Purdue Pharma, including the Sackler family, bear responsibility for the opioid crisis? Why or why not? If not, who else do you think is responsible? Explain your reasoning.

3. According to Brian Mann, what has made the Purdue Pharma bankruptcy case so difficult to settle? Do you think giving the Sackler family immunity from future opioid lawsuits in exchange billions of dollars for opioid addiction research and to support the families of victims of the opioid crisis is acceptable? Why or why not?

Chapter 4

1. Doctors can play a role in helping stop the opioid crisis. How do they suggest they can do this?
2. What are some of the ways in which the opioid crisis has changed since the beginning of the COVID-19 pandemic, as explained by Dennis Thompson? Overall, do you think the changes have had a positive or negative effect on controlling the opioid crisis? Explain your reasoning.
3. Would decriminalizing drugs and regulating drug trade have a positive impact on health and crime rates? Why or why not?

Organizations to Contact

The editors have compiled the following list of organizations concerned with the issues debated in this book. The descriptions are derived from materials provided by the organizations. All have publications or information available for interested readers. The list was compiled on the date of publication of the present volume; the information provided here may change. Be aware that many organizations take several weeks or longer to respond to inquiries, so allow as much time as possible.

Allied Against Opioid Abuse (AAOA)

email: info@againstopioidabuse.org
website: https://againstopioidabuse.org

Allied Against Opioid Use (AAOA) is an American education and awareness initiative to help prevent the abuse and misuse of prescription opioids. The organization collaborates with partners in pharmaceutical supply chains and public health and health-care organizations. Its website includes facts and data on opioid abuse.

American Medical Association (AMA)

AMA Plaza
330 N Wabash Ave., Suite 39300
Chicago, IL 60611-5885
(312) 464-4782
website: www.ama-assn.org

The American Medical Association (AMA) is a professional organization and lobbying group of physicians and medical students. In recent years, one of its top priorities has been helping to end the opioid crisis, with an emphasis on overdose prevention and treatment. Its website contains information about the steps physicians are taking to help curb opioid overdoses and information about treating opioid addiction.

Canadian Centre on Substance Use and Addiction (CCSA)

75 Albert Street, Suite 500
Ottawa, ON
K19 5E7
CANADA
1 (833) 235-4048
website: www.ccsa.ca

The Canadian Centre on Substance Use and Addiction (CCSA) was created through an Act of Parliament in 1988 as a non-governmental organization that aims to provide national leadership on substance use and solutions to drug and alcohol-related issues. Its website features data, information on different substances and types of addiction, and publications.

Centre for Addiction and Mental Health (CAMH)

1051 Queen St. West
Toronto, ON
M6J 1H3
CANADA
(416) 535-8501
website: www.camh.ca

The Centre for Addiction and Mental Health (CAMH) is Canada's largest mental health teaching hospital and one of the world's leading research centers in the field of addiction and mental health. It has a staff of over 3,000 physicians, researchers, clinicians, educators, and supporting staff. Its website contains health information, research materials, and information for Canadian patients in need of treatment.

Drug Enforcement Administration (DEA)

8701 Morrissette Drive
Springfield, VA 22152
(202) 307-1000
email: DEA.Public.Affairs@dea.gov
website: www.dea.gov

The Drug Enforcement Administration is a U.S. federal enforcement agency that is part of the Department of Justice. Its purpose is to prevent drug trafficking and distribution in the U.S. Its website features fact sheets about drugs, resources for recovering from addiction, and data and statistics related to their work.

National Institute on Drug Abuse (NIDA)

Office of Science Policy and Communication
3WFN MSC 6024
301 North Stonestreet Ave.
Bethesda, MD 20892
(301) 443-6441
website: https://nida.nih.gov

The National Institute on Drug Abuse (NIDA) is a U.S. federal government research institute that researches the causes and consequences of drug use and addiction. Its website features information about its research, infographics related to drug abuse and addiction, and the latest news on the topic.

Opioid Response Network (ORN)

(401) 270-5900
email: orn@aaap.org
website: https://opioidresponsenetwork.org

The Opioid Response Network (ORN) was created through a grant from the Substance Abuse and Mental Health Administration (SAMSHA) and in collaboration with the American Academy of Addiction Psychiatry (AAAP) and the Addiction Technology Transfer Center Network. ORN provides training and technical assistance in opioid treatment and response through local experts located throughout the U.S. Its website features information about the work they do, lessons learned, and educational resources.

Starts with One

Division of Behavioral Health and Recovery
P.O. Box 45330
Olympia, WA 98504-5330
(866) 789-1511
email: prevention@hca.wa.gov
website: https://getthefactsrx.com

The Starts with One campaign is a project of the Washington State Health Care Authority that was created to inform and educate young adults, their parents, and older adults about the dangers of prescription drug abuse. Its website includes opioid facts, information about safe storage and disposal of prescription opioids, and resources for starting a conversation on prescription opioid misuse.

Substance Abuse and Mental Health Services Administration (SAMHSA)

5600 Fishers Lane
Rockville, MD 20857
(877) 726-4727
website: www.samhsa.gov

The Substance Abuse and Mental Health Services Administration is a branch of the U.S. Department of Health and Human Services. Its aim is to improve the quality and availability of treatment for conditions related to mental health and substance abuse. Its website features information about finding treatment and health as well as data, news, and publications related to substance abuse and mental health.

Tribal Opioid Response Resource Toolkit

National Indian Health Board
910 Pennsylvania Ave., SE
Washington, DC 20003
(202) 507-4081
email: cwheeler@nihb.org
website: www.nihb.org/behavioral_health/tribal_opioid_response_resources.php

The Tribal Opioid Response Resource Toolkit is a project of the National Indian Health Board which is a nonprofit organization that provides policy analysis and advocacy on American Indian and Alaska Native health and public health services. Its resources toolkit contains data and information on addressing the opioid crisis in tribal communities.

Bibliography of Books

Barbara Andraka-Christou. *The Opioid Fix: America's Addiction Crisis and the Solution They Don't Want You to Have.* Baltimore, MD: Johns Hopkins University Press, 2020.

M. M. Eboch, ed. *Prescription Drugs* (Introducing Issues with Opposing Viewpoints). New York, NY: Greenhaven Publishing, 2020.

John H. Halpern and David Blistein. *Opium: How an Ancient Flower Shaped and Poisoned Our World.* New York, NY: Hachette Books, 2020.

Ryan Hampton. *Unsettled: How the Purdue Pharma Bankruptcy Failed the Victims of the American Overdose Crisis.* New York, NY: St. Martin's Press, 2021.

Kojo Koram. *The War on Drugs and the Global Colour Line.* London, UK: Pluto Press, 2019.

Barbara Krasner, ed. *Harm Reduction: Public Health Strategies* (Opposing Viewpoints). New York, NY: Greenhaven Publishing, 2019.

Beth Macy. *Dopesick: Dealers, Doctors, and the Drug Company that Addicted America.* Reprint ed. New York, NY: Back Bay Books, 2019.

Chris McGreal. *American Overdose: The Opioid Crisis in Three Acts.* New York, NY: PublicAffairs, 2018.

Barry Meier. *Pain Killer: An Empire of Deceit and the Origin of America's Opioid Crisis.* 2nd ed. New York, NY: Random House, 2018.

Nadra Nittle, ed. *America's Mental Health Crisis* (Current Controversies). New York, NY: Greenhaven Publishing, 2019.

Sam Quinones. *The Least of Us: True Tales of America and Hope in the Time of Fentanyl and Meth*. New York, NY: Bloomsbury Publishing, 2021.

Patrick Radden Keefe. *Empire of Pain: The Secret History of the Sackler Dynasty*. New York, NY: Doubleday, 2021.

Travis Rieder. *In Pain: A Bioethicist's Personal Struggle with Opioids*. New York, NY: Harper Paperbacks, 2020.

Jonathan D. Rosen. *The U.S. War on Drugs at Home and Abroad*. London, UK: Palgrave Macmillan, 2021.

Michael Rosino. *Debating the Drug War: Race, Politics, and the Media* (Framing 21st Century Social Issues). New York, NY: Routledge, 2021.

Maia Szalavitz. *Undoing Drugs: The Untold Story of Harm Reduction and the Future of Addiction*. New York, NY: Hachette Go, 2021.

Brett Ann Stanciu. *Unstitched: My Journey to Understand Opioid Addiction and How People and Communities Can Heal*. Hanover, NH: Steerforth Press, 2021.

Ben Westhoff. *Fentanyl, Inc.: How Rogue Chemists Are Creating the Deadliest Wave of the Opioid Epidemic*. New York, NY: Grove Atlantic, 2019.

Index